The Herbal Remedies & Natural Medicine Bible

© Copyright 2023 by Triya Nanavati

This document is geared towards providing exact and reliable information with regards to the topic and issue covered. The publication is sold with the idea that the publisher is not required to render accounting, officially permitted, or otherwise, qualified services. If advice is necessary, legal or professional, a practiced individual in the profession should be ordered.

From a Declaration of Principles which was accepted and approved equally by a Committee of the American Bar Association and a Committee of Publishers and Associations.

In no way is it legal to reproduce, duplicate, or transmit any part of this document in either electronic means or in printed format. Recording of this publication is strictly prohibited and any storage of this document is not allowed unless with written permission from the publisher.

All rights reserved.

The information provided herein is stated to be truthful and consistent, in that any liability, in terms of inattention or otherwise, by any usage or abuse of any policies, processes, or directions contained within is the solitary and utter responsibility of the recipient reader. Under no circumstances will any legal responsibility or blame be held against the publisher for any reparation, damages, or monetary loss due to the information herein, either directly or indirectly.

Copyright © 2023 by Triya Nanavati
All rights reserved. No part of this book may be reproduced, scanned, or distributed in any printed or electronic form without permission.

First Edition: June 2023

Cover: Illustration made by Mary F.

Printed in the United States of America

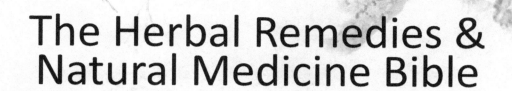

The Herbal Remedies & Natural Medicine Bible

The Comprehensive Guide to Cultivate, Grow and Harvest Healing Herbs and Plants to Prepare Infusions, Essentials Oils and Natural Antibiotics

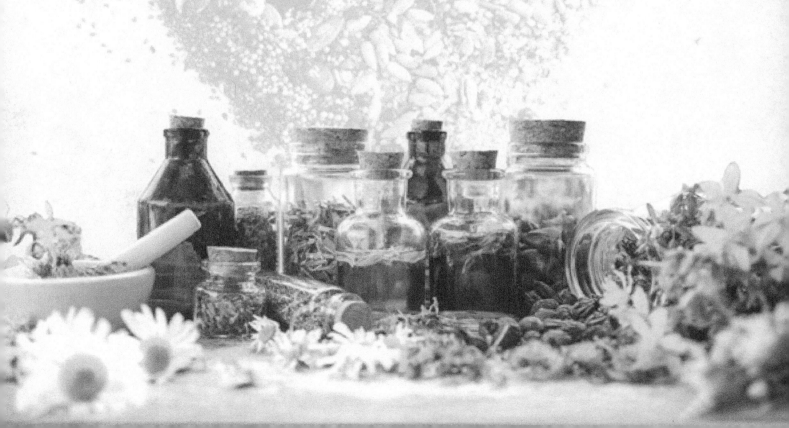

Triya Nanavati

TABLE OF CONTENTS

PART 1 -
ORIGIN OF HERBAL HEALING .... Page 1

PART 2 -
NATURAL MEDICINAL PRACTICE .... « 5

PART 3 -
HOW EFFECTIVE IS MEDICINAL HERBS .... « 9

PART 4 -
DIFFERENT FORMS OF MEDICINAL HERBS .... « 13

PART 5 -
HERBS TO BE CONSUMED AND AVOIDED .... « 19

PART 6 -
HERBAL TREATMENT FOR ANXIETY .... « 45

PART 7 -
MEDICINAL HERBS TO BOOST THE IMMUNE SYSTEM .... « 47

PART 8 -
MEDICINAL HERBS TO LOSE WEIGHT .... « 51

PART 9 -
MEDICINAL HERBS TO CURE INSOMNIA .... « 53

PART 10 -
MEDICINAL HERBS TO FIGHT INFLAMMATION .... « 59

PART 11 -
HERBAL TREATMENT TO RELIEVE STRESS .... « 61

PART 12 -
MEDICINAL HERBS FOR HIGH BLOOD PRESSURE .... « 63

PART 13 -
HERBS FOR ARTHRITIS .... « 65

PART 14 -
HERBS FOR OTHER COMMON DISEASES .... « 67

PART 15 -
    MEDICINAL HERBS IN ORIENTAL TRADITION.................................... Page 71

PART 16 -
    FRESH HERBS AND DRIED HERB.. « 77

PART 17 -
    ESSENTIAL OILS.. « 83

CONCLUSION - .... « 87

BONUS 1 -
    TIPS FOR GROWING HERBS... « 89

BONUS 2 -
    THE 9 APHRODISIAC HERBS... « 95

BONUS 3 -
    TYPES OF HERBS TO BE AVOIDED.. « 105

BONUS 4 -
    HERBS FOR FACIAL CARE.. « 109

AUTHOR BIO -
    TRIYA NANAVATI.. « 111

Dedicated to all my friends and to all the people
who gave me their help.
Thanks a lot
Thanks to all of you for your confidence
in my qualities and what I do.
Triya Nanavati

PART 1

ORIGIN OF HERBAL HEALING

It has been practiced for thousands of years all throughout the world to treat illnesses with herbs. The majority of these documents are from China, Egypt, and Greece, the country where Hippocrates was born. He is known as the "Father of Medicine" and is credited with stating, "Let the meal be your medicine."

A true, acknowledged, and valued contribution to the treatment of illnesses, injuries, and disease has been made for a long time by herbal treatments and medicine.

The first "herbalists" were actually people who lived in the area and had a profound awareness of the healing properties of various plants and herbs. Such knowledge was acquired and transmitted over many years by word of mouth and came from a society that was not constrained by the naming of active components, chemical enhancers, complex formulations, and patents.

When the use of herbal medicine was associated with witchcraft, black magic, and the occult at a later point in our world's history, there was widespread mistrust, misunderstanding, and a legitimate fear of the unknown. Tragically, as a result of these animosities, the majority of innocent individuals suffered persecution and were burned at the stake for being witches.

But in more recent times, it appears that our community is pleading for a change to more alternative, non-invasive, holistic, and organic remedies. Because of this, the use of medical plants and related herbal therapies has been prevalent for a long time. Herbal medicines are making a comeback as we search for more natural and less clinical solutions.

Long before the ancient era, plants were employed for healing purposes. Chinese teachings and ancient Unani writings on Egyptian papyrus describe how to use plants.

There is proof that herbal medicine has been used by Unani Hakims, Indian Vaids, and European and Mediterranean cultures for more than 4000 years. In addition to other ancient medical ideologies like

Unani, Ayurveda, and Chinese medicine, indigenous societies in Persia, Arabia, India, Africa, and America have utilized plants for medicinal rites.

India has long been regarded as one of the most abundant repositories of medicinal herbs among ancient civilizations. India's forests are the world's greatest reservoir of a variety of aromatic and medicinal plants, which are mostly harvested as raw materials for the production of pharmaceuticals and scented products. In India's AYUSH systems, some 8,000 herbal treatments have been formalized. The four main categories of indigenous medicines are Ayurveda, Unani, Siddha, and folk (tribal) remedies. The most advanced and commonly used of these practices in India are Ayurveda and Unani

80 percent of people worldwide currently rely on herbal medications for some aspect of their basic healthcare requirements, according to the WHO (World Health Organization). Around 21,000 plant species may be utilized as therapeutic herbs, according to the WHO.

Vegetables and plant extracts are the primary sources of health care for more than three-quarters of the world's population, according to current studies. More than 30% of all plant species have been utilized for medicinal purposes at some stage. According to estimates, plant-based pharmaceuticals make up up to 25% of all drugs in affluent nations like the United States, while they make up up to 80% of all drugs in nations with rapid economic growth like India and China. Therefore, countries like India place a much greater emphasis on the economic value of medicinal plants than does the rest of the globe. Two-thirds of the crops used in modern medicine come from these nations, and traditional medicine is the mainstay of the health care system for the underprivileged.

Treatment with medicinal plants is well known to be highly beneficial because the adverse effects are either nonexistent or minimal. The biggest benefit of these treatments is that they are in sync with nature. The bright side is that pharmaceutical treatments are appropriate for people of all ages and genders.

According to ancient writers, plants can only be used as alternatives to a number of illnesses and health issues. They conducted a comprehensive investigation into the matter and conducted tests to determine the accuracy of their conclusions on the efficacy of various therapeutic plants. The majority of the medications created in this way had no adverse effects or responses. Because of this, herbal medicine is becoming more popular worldwide. These herbal plants provide acceptable methods for the detection of several internal ailments that are otherwise thought to be incurable.

Numerous common ailments may be cured with plants used in medicine, including aloe, tulsi, neem, turmeric, and ginger. Many areas of the nation view them as natural treatments. Many consumers reportedly utilize basil (also known as tulsi) to make black tea, puja, medications, and other items for everyday usage.

A number of plants are used by people in many regions of the world to honor their rulers as lucky charms. Now that people are aware of the use of herbs in medicine, many of them are beginning to grow tulsi and other healing plants in their backyard gardens.

It is well recognized that medicinal plants are a rich supply of components that may be utilized to make either pharmacopoeial, non-pharmaceutical, or artificial medications. This is partially due to the crucial role that these crops have played in the development of human cultures all across the world. On the other hand, certain plants are recognized as being an important source of nourishment and are consequently recognized for their medicinal benefits. These plants include ones that produce ginger, green tea, walnuts, aloe, pepper, turmeric, and others. It is well recognized that many plants and their extracts constitute a significant source of the active chemicals included in products like aspirin and toothpaste. Herbs are utilized not just for medical purposes but also for natural coloring, pest control, meat, perfume, tea, and other things. Many nations employ various medical plants and herbs to keep bees, rats, and other pests out of homes and businesses while allowing them to flee. These days, medicinal plants are significant sources for the manufacture of pharmaceuticals.

Traditional medical practitioners have had great success prescribing herbs to cure common illnesses including vomiting, constipation, diabetes, low sperm count, dysentery, and hindered penile erection, as well as masses, powdered lips, irregular menstruation, bronchial asthma, leucorrhoea, and fever.

Although the use of herbal medicine has significantly increased over the past 20 years, there is still a dearth of research data in this field. However, the WHO has released three collections of WHO monographs on certain medicinal plants since 1999.

PART 2

NATURAL MEDICINAL PRACTICE

When we talk about "herbology" or "herbal medicine," we're talking about the many plant species that are used in herbalism. This includes researching and using plants for medicinal purposes.

The words "herb" and "herbe," which are pre-French words, are derived from the Latin word "herba" and the French word "herbe." Today, any component of the plant, including the berries, seeds, base, bark, vine, leaves, stigma, or heart of the plant, might be referred to as a "herb". The term "herb" was used to refer only to non-woody plants, such as those derived from shrubs, trees, and roots. Additionally, these medicinal plants are used in food, medicine, flavonoids, perfume, and a few religious rites.

Traditional therapeutic concepts are commonly applied, according to several accounts. A growing emphasis has been placed on using plant materials as a source for pharmaceutical ingredients for a variety of human illnesses due to a number of factors, including the increase in population, the scarcity of medications, their prohibitive cost, their side effects when compared to natural remedies, and the development of immunity to infectious diseases that are more frequently encountered.

The practice of using natural or medicinal plants to treat illness is known as herbal therapy or herbalism. Herbal medicine is meant to support the body's ability to heal itself via homeostasis rather than be a standalone therapy for a disorder.

The body has to be in a state where pollutants are eliminated and the organs are functioning within the body's environment in order for it to calm down or spontaneously begin the self-healing process. Homeostasis is the name given to this state.

Some of the major advantages of using medicinal herbs and herbal cleansing include their relatively low production and use costs, the fact that they are grown and produced organically, and the fact that because these treatments are derived from the world of plants, the possibility of side effects is decreased because the body is designed to tolerate them. Herbal medicine used by a qualified psychologist or physician involves a small risk.

Natural medicine is not only about drinking and eating Skittles; however, certain places must exercise caution while opting to partake in these alternative therapies.

Although herbs are naturally occurring, they can nonetheless be harmful to you. Always seek the counsel of a qualified and reputable herbal medicine practitioner when treating serious or persistent medical conditions. The secret to success here is dose.

Despite what your friends, family, or coworkers may well intend, avoid using any herbs as over-the-counter treatments or acting upon any advice offered to you without adequate information to serve as a guide. It's also a beautiful idea to be aware of how the medication you decide to take really eases the condition you're managing.

Learn all there is to know about the medicinal herbs you are cultivating, including their botanical names, any known risks, how precisely they grow, and how they emerge and flower if you plan to cultivate them yourself. Make sure they are appropriately labeled when buying seedlings and that you are completely aware of what you are acquiring if you are just starting out on your herb adventure and are unaware of what your herb plants are. For the greatest results, try mixing many different types of herbs that have comparable capabilities rather than putting all your eggs in one single herb.

Please be aware that using herbal medicine properly is absolutely safe and a terrific alternative strategy and activity. For your convenience, a short introduction to herbal medicine and its application has been provided.

The dose determines whether a substance is a poison or a treatment, claimed Paracelsus in the 16th century. Do you really possess a "great herb garden"? Medicinal plants are the best bioresource for traditional treatments, modern pharmaceuticals, nutraceuticals, nutritional supplements, folk remedies, and chemical agents for synthetic drugs.

Herbal medicines have been used in traditional and ethnomedical practices for a very long time. This section examines crop genomics, evolution, and phylogeny's current conditions and anticipated advances. These diverse fields at the interface of phytochemistry and plant biology address a wide range of issues, including the evolution and systematics of medicinal plant genomes, the genesis and inheritance of plant genotypes, the inheritance of metabolic phenotypes, the relationship between the environment and the genomes of medicinal plants, and the relationship between genomic diversity and metabolite diversity, among others. Modern genomic technologies may be applied to agricultural plants as well as traditional medicinal plants to hasten the breeding of medical plants and produce a living plant with therapeutic components.

The application of genetic phylogenomics and phylogenomics in predicting chemical diversity and bioprospecting is highlighted by the creation and production of medications derived from natural materials.

Representative case studies of the medicinal plant genome, phylogeny, and evolution were provided in order to highlight the extension of information pedigree and the paradigm shift to omics-based techniques. These case studies assist both the molecular breeding of medicinal plants and the sustainable use of plant pharmacological assets by updating our understanding of the evolution of plant genomes.

Over time, African medicinal plants have assimilated into the civilization of the continent and are now largely regarded as a reflection of its rich scientific and cultural heritage. The rising demand for medicinal plant components has reignited the pharmaceutical industry's interest in creating herbal nutritional supplements, herbal cosmetics, and herbal health care formulas. Therefore, in addition to meeting medical and social demands, medicinal plants are important commercially in Africa.

Sales of goods manufactured from medicinal plants have expanded into new local and global markets and resulted in significant financial advantages. This book will describe the therapeutic plants utilized in different African countries and examine how local enterprises employ them. The marketing and distribution of medicinal plants in local African markets mostly focuses on broad trends, patterns, and circumstances that are seen often.

Triya Nanavati

PART 3

HOW EFFECTIVE IS MEDICINAL HERBS

Due to their extensive long-term use in so many diverse contexts, citizens all over the world are aware of what medicinal plants are and are in awe of their miracles. Because they are ideal flavor enhancers and spices for cooking. The flowery smells of the herbal plants are also utilized in various relaxing and pressure-reduction techniques. These are not the only options, though; several plants may also be used to cure a range of human ailments and disorders.

People who have lived on the planet have long been aware of the medical benefits of plants. Additionally, a number of incidents involving the use of plants to treat people's ailments are mentioned in biblical tales. The use of therapeutic plants has evolved recently along with technological development.

A number of different medical plant kinds are currently being made into pills, syrups, tablets, and dietary supplements. However, the majority of conventional techniques are still employed by both young and elderly individuals to treat pain, sores, and other ailments.

Herbs are valued for their therapeutic benefits and work in a few straightforward yet effective ways. The traditional methods for gathering therapeutic plants include boiling, beating, grilling, and mincing. Even some medications work effectively when administered directly to the wound or to the portion of the body that is afflicted.

Whatever approach you use, the surprising effects of these therapeutic plants will leave you in awe. By employing these herbs, the painful body parts may be soothed, sweating and spasms can be prevented, body pains can be reduced, and pressure can be released. Herbs may be used to treat everything from allergies to blood flow abnormalities. Yes, using herbs has a number of advantages, and more advantages are probably to come as more study is done.

Medical plants have earned their proper position in the field of contemporary medicine throughout the years. In truth, before they developed their own approach to treating patients, medical practitioners have always been concerned with plants. Additionally, herbal essences and oils have frequently been combined with other medicinal components to create convenient medications.

Recently, it has been discovered that certain plants may be used to cure deadly ailments, including hypertension, cardiovascular, respiratory, and digestive system issues. As a result, medicinal plants and medications work effectively together.

The best thing about therapeutic herbs is that they are inexpensive and widely accessible. Now, illnesses may be cured even for individuals who cannot afford expert medical care. You'll be able to uncover a natural route to health by just looking around. From a comfort perspective, drugs made from other substances are more expensive than tablets and capsules made from plants.

The best part is that there is a lower possibility of negative effects with herbal medicine. The use of medicinal herbs is a quick answer to everyone's expanding medical demands, provided you have the right information and training.

Many naturally occurring compounds (constituents) found in herbs have some sort of biological action. Herbs function similarly to several pharmaceutical medications. Some medications are still produced using plants today. For instance, the bark of the cinchona tree is used to extract the malaria drug quinine, while the opium poppy is used to make morphine, a painkiller.

However, in order to ensure that the crop's nutritional balance is maintained, European herbalists concur that herbs should be used in their whole form. They discovered that treating serious, reoccurring ailments with natural therapies had the best results. Herbal remedies are often not available as quick fixes.

Herbalists frequently assert that some ailments may be effectively treated by plants without the unfavorable side effects frequently associated with conventional medical treatments. But it's important to keep in mind that certain herbs are quite potent and might have harmful side effects if taken incorrectly.

Some herbs may also have an impact on how the body reacts to over-the-counter and prescription medications, either by reducing or amplifying their effects.

Before taking herbal medicines, feel free to speak with a fully qualified herbalist. Herbalists have received training in how to blend treatments, as well as how much and how long to use them for various ailments and outcomes. Additionally, we aim to treat the individual as a whole, utilizing entire herbal remedies to strengthen the body's natural ability to heal itself. In addition to treating a person's illness or ailment, herbs are chosen to match each individual.

Herbal Supplements

Herbal products, botanicals, or phytomedicines are made from plants or botanicals that are used to heal illnesses or preserve food. A plant-based treatment used just for internal consumption is known as an herbal alternative.

The majority of generic and over-the-counter medications are likewise made from plant materials, but they only have pure components and are FDA-regulated. Whole plants or plant components can be found in herbal supplements.

Herbal supplements can be eaten as pills, powders, tinctures, or combined into tea. They can also be applied topically as gels, lotions, or creams, or added to bathwater. They come in all different shapes and sizes.

Herbal supplements have been used for thousands of years. These days, American customers frequently take herbal supplements. But not everyone will enjoy them. The use of herbal supplements is still debatable since they are not closely regulated by the FDA or other regulatory agencies. It is advisable to discuss any illnesses or conditions you may have with a doctor, who can also advise you on the use of herbal supplements.

Herbal supplements and the FDA Herbal supplements are meat, according to the FDA, not medications. As a result, they are not held to the same screening, processing, and branding requirements and laws as medications.

You may now view stickers that explain how various bodily functions will be impacted by medications. However, the labeling of herbal supplements cannot mention the treatment of certain medical diseases. This is due to the fact that herbal treatments do not conflict with clinical research or meet the same quality criteria as typical over-the-counter or prescription medications.

Contrary to medicines, herbal supplements are not anticipated to be standardized to assure batch-to-batch stability. Even though most businesses use the same term on their product tags, the meaning varies depending on which provider is used.

PART 4

DIFFERENT FORMS OF MEDICINAL HERBS

Herbal medicines are created in a variety of consistent forms across traditional herbal medicine programs. These forms often change based on the plant utilized and, occasionally, the ailment being treated. Some of these techniques, which will be covered in more detail in this chapter, are infusions (hot teas), decoctions (cooked teas), tinctures (alcohol and water extracts), and macerations (cold soaking). In contrast to others, medicinal practitioners or shamans often employ the same methods in traditional Indigenous therapeutic systems. Others include treating plants in hot baths (in which the patient is submerged or bathed), inhaling plant powder (like snuff), inhaling the steam from various herbal plants that have been cooked in hot water, and even aromatherapy. Here, a few of the techniques will be covered in more detail.

Concoctions

These are aqueous solutions that have been submerged or boiled in liquid for different plant sections for a predetermined amount of time. To ensure a thorough extraction, it is steeped for three days before usage if it is drained rather than boiled for 15–20 minutes. The mixture can also be made into a soup known as "aseje" in traditional medicine by cooking it with plant pieces. These soups may be made by adding a variety of additional ingredients, and they can be made to last a whole day.

Decoctions

Decoctions are aqueous preparations of plant components that have been cooked in water for 15 to 20 minutes until the water volume has been reduced by half. Decoctions are made by chopping plant components into tiny bits and soaking them in a large amount of water in an earthenware pail (palayok). After adding enough liquid to cover the plant parts in the bowl, the mixture should be cooked until the water content is cut in half. The boiling preparation is stored for two to three days by filtering, cooling, and refrigerating it.

Powerful concoctions Strong decoctions are made in one of two ways, depending on the type of plant material utilized. The combination should first be boiled for a longer period of time. This is frequently shown while working with larger woody bark fragments. Sometimes melting, softening, and removing bigger chunks require a longer boiling period of up to two hours. Instead, the decoction is produced as above (for a boiling time of 20 minutes), then the herb is left to soak overnight before being filtered if smaller woody portions are employed but a stronger solution is required. To get the most decoction from the chopped herb pieces during extraction, they are forced into the sieve.

Dry decoctions

Dry decoctions were created in Japan in the 1950s and are now a widely used herbal method in that country as well as Taiwan, the US, and Europe. Large quantities of herb formulations are made into decoctions (in big tanks), and the fluid is then extracted from the solid residue to generate dry decoctions. A solution is then produced by evaporating the water using heat and vacuumd herbal method in that country as well as Taiwan, the US, and Europe. Large quantities of herb formulations are made into decoctions (in big tanks), and the fluid is then extracted from the solid residue to generate dry decoctions. A solution is then produced by evaporating the water using heat and vacuum. The surplus moisture is subsequently removed from the solution using a spray dryer coupled with a powder carrier (often starch or washed, crushed, or herb dregs), resulting in a dry powder.

Infusions

Infusions are created using either fresh or dried herbs, much like when making tea. Plant parts are submerged in hot water for 10 minutes and allowed to stand. After filtering the tea, you can enjoy it hot or cold. Just for a single day's use.

Drugs

Similar to brewing tea, infusions can be made using fresh or dried herbs. Plant components are dipped for ten minutes in hot water and then let stand. You may drink the tea hot or cold after filtering it. only for one usage each day.

Powder

The traditional Yoruba inhabitants refer to this dish as "Agunmu." Using a mortar and pestle, the well-dried plant product is crushed and pounded into a chic, homogeneous powder. This is the most common and simple technique for manufacturing herbal medicines. To ensure higher solubility, the dust is confined in sterile containers and should be as tiny as feasible. While native healers in Oromo, Southwest Ethiopia's Gambi area, employed a variety of techniques to make traditional herbal remedies, powdering and pounding are the two techniques that are most frequently used.

Tinctures

Alcoholic decoction is another name for this mixture. The plant components are either fresh or dried and kept at 40–60% alcohol proof for the manufacturing of tinctures. One piece of the herb is combined with five sections of distilled liquor to make the preparation, which is then put in an airtight container. At least once each day, the solution is shaken or stirred. Extracts from alcoholic decoctions keep the vital components as long as feasible. In an airtight glass container, the extract is treated after filtering. Usually, five to twenty drops are administered either topically or straight into the beverage. This is frequently accomplished by boiling the liquor in water with your preferred herbs. The mixture would then be compressed and tightly sealed into a jar. The remaining solution can be utilized to create the ointment after two weeks of use.

Tablets

Valuable herbs are ground and properly combined. A portion of the dried product's content may be decocted into a thick condensed liquid and then blended with additional powdered ingredients when small tablets with a high drug concentration are needed. When making the tablet, enough starch or rice paste is added to the mixture before being briskly shaken and kneaded by hands. With the assistance of a cheap tablet, which can be constructed of wood or iron, large globular tablets are created from a material that is kneaded into a paste-like consistency.

Syrup

A specified quantity of cane sugar is dissolved in a certain volume of boiling water until the sugar is completely dissolved in the water for this crucial therapy for kids and babies. The desired herb is cooked, decanted, and then poured into water. The resulting extract is added to the prepared cane sugar syrup in a ratio of 1:1. Typically, 1 ml of the decoction fluid contains 1 g of the extracted medication. If the syrup is not going to be used, a significant amount of fungicide should be preserved as benzoic acid for further processing.

Poultice

It may also be created by crushing and grinding the necessary plant material, whether it is dry or fresh (fresh is preferred), with a little heat, oil, or honey. The resultant paste is then applied or bonded to the afflicted region using a square of clean linen or a banana trunk. However, pulp can also be made by boiling the crushed crop.

Compresses

Usually, they are softer than seeds. A moist cloth or banana trunk is soaked in an infusion or decoction and applied to the afflicted regions.

Juices

Juice is produced by pressing fruit pieces or by crushing fresh plant material and sifting it through a fine mesh sieve.

Using Herbal Medicine as First Aid

Natural first aid techniques sometimes involve the use of medicinal plants, such as applying lavender oil to burns or rubbing dock leaves on nettle stings. In both emergency and non-emergency situations, herbs are used to treat a wide range of medical problems, from insect stings and nausea to serious wounds.

Even though a large portion of this technique has been abandoned in contemporary times, using native plants to treat minor illnesses is once again gaining popularity. The majority of herbalists provide basic seminars where you can learn more about anything from plant identification to treatments.

There are several instances where pharmaceutical medications and plants work effectively together.

Nevertheless, there might occasionally be bad things that happen. Some plants should not be used with certain medications. Your herbalist can provide advice in any situation since they are educated to know which drugs to use safely.

How long will herbal therapy last?

Since there are so many factors that will affect how long therapy lasts, there is no conclusive solution. Our bodies recover at different speeds, and our biological makeup is as distinct as our medical history.

Disease, disease severity, and the type of treatment required are influencing variables. How long it has been in place, any prior medical history, any medical background, and the present state of your health Once they have given you a thorough account of the incident, the herbalist might be able to give you a recommendation that is correct. It is crucial to regularly evaluate progress and to change herbal drugs as needed over time.

Compared to pharmaceutical medications, herbal medicine may occasionally take longer before it begins to have the intended impact. To uncover the condition's underlying cause, it takes a calm and helpful approach, which may be what ultimately leads to more lasting effects. In addition, adverse effects are uncommon when medication is used as directed.

While the aforementioned is true for chronic conditions, the correct amount of herbs can deliver quick effects. In first-aid situations, health herbalists commonly address serious issues within a few hours or days.

Professional guidance is necessary since the use of herbs and their correct administration are crucial to their safety and effectiveness.

PART 5

HERBS TO BE CONSUMED AND AVOIDED

It is suggested that we be aware of any herbs we want to consume. Not all substances should be digested because some might seriously harm our health. For this reason, some therapeutic herbs should only be applied topically.

It is essential that the people in charge of our care be completely aware of the prescriptions you are taking, including any counterproducts, dietary supplements, or herbal remedies.

Aloe Vera

Numerous medical benefits may be derived from the aloe vera plant, which has been utilized for this purpose for many years. Once established, the aloe plant is quite simple to reproduce and doesn't require daily or even weekly watering. Because of this, the aloe plant is a fantastic choice for people who occasionally travel or for those who might forget to water it. Take a look at some of this herb's previously described therapeutic properties.

Medicinal Uses:

- Burns Psoriasis Diabetes Colitis Immune
- Aid Anti-inflammatory
- Body toner
- Wound Healer
- Aloe gel can be use for burns

Aloe should be used most often to treat burns, wounds, and skin disorders. Aloe plants are a great addition to your natural first aid kit because of how easy they are to grow. The aloe vera leaf's true healing power is found in its gel, which may be obtained by simply taking a knife to the leaf's thick skin on the exterior.

Because you're essentially filling the seed, the component is a transparent interior fluid that is sometimes referred to as the inner filet. Hold the injured area under cool water for approximately ten minutes to treat small burns before applying the aloe gel. Apply the solution to all wounds and skin issues repeatedly each day. Start taking one tablespoon of aloe gel each day if you're using it to lower your blood sugar levels, and when taking it orally, make sure the gel is devoid of aloin.

Attention: Avoid applying aloe vera to any open wounds when using the herb. Likewise, exercise caution while touching the seeds. You should use the clear gel component, as I said before, to remove the oozing yellow sap. When eating aloe gel orally, you should be aware of this yellow fluid, even if it's not a huge concern when applied to the body. The laxative properties of the yellow sap, known as aloin, can lead to electrolyte depletion and dependence on regular bowel movements if taken for an extended length of time.

Basil Herbs

Basil Basil has a position in herbal medicine in addition to being a great plant for cooking. I do enjoy basil plants since they are easy to nurture; all you have to do is make sure to give them some regular watering. It is a very fragrant plant with a flavor and scent that are somewhat alcoholic. Basil can be cloned, which is a great thing I've discovered you can do with it.

Finding the plant you wish to reproduce (the parent plant) and trimming it 3–4 inches down from the top of the stem are really not that difficult. You must ensure that the cut you make is far above a node. Here, the plant attaches to the stem body and develops new growth. In order to leave a stem with 4-6 leaves on top, simply remove the bottom leaves of the cut. Just plant a new basil clone in some earth after placing the cut into a small dish of water and waiting for the roots to sprout. I've discovered that applying honey and a rooting hormone to the stem's outside edge really aids in accelerating plant development. Let's look at the qualities of the basil plant that we may employ. As I indicated earlier, basil has a place in traditional medicine.

Uses :

- Serve as an antibacterial
- Strong sedative
- Relieves pain Bites and Stings

Basil has a very significant impact on the digestive system, as you might expect from a plant of its kind, and is consequently excellent for treating indigestion, bloating, and nausea. I'd advise taking 2-4 grams of basil orally daily when using it to treat these symptoms. Basil may also be used to treat bug bites and stings; simply crush the leaves and apply the fluids to the region that has been harmed.

Basil performs extremely well as a pesticide, so it tends to kill insects, so if you get bitten or stung, make sure you apply the juice to your body in the same way.

Calendula Herbal

Calendula is different from the ordinary marigold that is frequently seen in gardens and is also known as pot marigold or poet's marigold. Calendula is safe to consume, and it smells far less than regular marigolds. The calendula plant was most frequently employed in England's stews, syrups, and bread throughout the Middle Ages.

Calendula is the ideal herb to cultivate since it is simple to start from seed and adapts to a variety of growth environments. The plant may be found in countless gardens from subarctic to tropical climates all over the world. Let's now examine the main medical applications that make calendula such a valuable plant.

Medicinal Uses:

- Anti-fungal
- Anti-inflammatory
- Wound Aid Antimicrobial
- Blood Moisturizer

Calendula ointment The most common uses for the calendula plant are in creams, lotions, ointments, and soaps. For millennia, calendula has been used to heal small injuries and skin diseases. The plant calendula can be administered orally to treat fever, stomach distress, and ulcers. The calendula plant is frequently used in medical settings to heal small wounds, burns, insect bites, and other conditions.

To aid with these digestive issues, it is suggested that you consume 3-5 grams per day. Making tea or tinctures from the petals is a great approach to treating peptic ulcers and digestive disorders, especially if you're using it to treat gluten sensitivity.

Caution: Calendula should not be used if you have an allergy to any Asteraceae plant. Any topical application that might result in the production of a rash could cause you to develop a sensitivity.

Cayenne Pepper

Calendula cream The calendula plant is most frequently utilized in creams, lotions, ointments, and soaps. Calendula has been used for thousands of years to treat minor wounds and skin conditions. Calendula is a plant that may be used orally to cure ulcers, stomach discomfort, and fever. The calendula plant is widely used for minor injuries, burns, bug bites, and various ailments in medicinal settings. You should take in 3-5 grams daily to help with these digestive problems, according to the recommendation. If you're utilizing the petals to treat gluten sensitivity, making tea or tinctures from them is a fantastic way to cure peptic ulcers and other digestive issues. If you have an allergy to any Asteraceae plant, avoid using calendula. You might become sensitive to any topical application that could result in the appearance of a rash.

Medicinal Uses:

- Antiseptic
- Natural analgesic
- Prevent irritant Stimulant
- Relieves pressure Inflammation
- Nerve Pain

It is most frequently used as a cream, lotion, or salve to treat fibromyalgia-related joint and muscular pain, shingles, and inflammation. When taken orally, this has also been demonstrated to enhance breathing, lessen heartburn, and ease discomfort from cluster headaches. For nerve discomfort, apply a lotion containing 0.075% capsaicin 3–4 times a day. By using cream with a concentration of around 0.025 percent four times a day, you can manage pain-type arthritis. Cayenne can also take 6 to 8 weeks to start functioning, but if you're careful, it will eventually provide results. Cayenne-containing capsules are a convenient way to consume the spice orally. Cayenne pepper has occasionally been reported to decrease hunger and increase calorie burn; however, this impact is probably negligible overall.

Applying capsaicin to the skin can result in burning, stinging, redness, and even a rash. Usually, this rash is only irritation, and it will go away after the first few applications. You should stop taking it if the rash doesn't go away, since capsaicin allergies are possible.

Additionally, broken skin should not be exposed to capsaicin. If you operate with more focus, remember to use gloves. If you don't have gloves, be sure to fully clean your hands before making contact with your face.

Chamomile

Another wonderful plant with many applications is chamomile. Manzanilla is the Spanish name for this plant, and it's no joke that the Spanish call it that since it practically means "little fruit." When the petals and leaves are crushed, an apparent apple aroma is released. German chamomile and Roman or English chamomile are the two main species of chamomile. Both have comparable medicinal benefits, but the Roman or English kind has a stronger perfume. All types may be grown from seed with relative ease, and if they are allowed to go to seed naturally, you will be able to watch their growth the following year.

Medicinal uses:

- Digestive relief
- Mouth ulcers
- Eczema
- Anti-allergenic
- Anti-inflammatory
- Wound cure

How to use chamomile

It is highly popular as a beverage and simple to make.

Put 1 teaspoon of dried chamomile in 1 cup of boiling water. Give the tea 5-7 minutes to steep; the longer you let the tea sit, the stronger the calming effects will be. It is also possible to buy chamomile pills, which are a reasonably simple way to get the benefits of chamomile. Making your own chamomile topical cream is another excellent technique to lessen eczema symptoms, although studies have shown that chamomile cream and a modest dose of hydrocortisone cream have similar effects.

Attention: Although it happens rarely, people who experience adverse reactions to chamomile typically have severe ragweed allergies. However, chamomile is generally regarded as a very harmless plant.

Chickweed

In temperate and polar locations all around the world, chickweed is a perennial plant. The chickweed has an intriguing habit of sleeping at night, when the leaves fold in to protect the tender buds and shoots. Chickweed is a nice herb to add to salads because it is also regarded as being quite.

The entire plant can be utilized in herbal treatments, both fresh and dried. Let's now examine the main medical applications for which this plant is most well-known.

Medicinal Uses:

- Astringent Demulcent
- Alleviates Itchyness
- Cooling effect when applied to the skin

How to use Chickweed

The ability of chickweed to soothe irritated skin makes it a popular treatment for eczema, nettle rash, and insect bites.

Olive oil, chickweed, beeswax, and lavender scent may all be used to create a simple chickweed herb. The chickweed should be coarsely chopped and let to dry for about 24 hours. The next step is to combine the equal amount of chickweed with olive oil and cook the mixture for 20 seconds.

The mixture should then be placed in a metal dish that is hung over a water-filled metal dish. To prevent the mixture from getting too heated, bring it to a boil in the bottom dish without letting the bottom of the top dish touch the water. Regularly stir the mixture, and then strain it through a cheese cloth. Instead, melt the beeswax and add the infused oil, mix to blend, and then extract using the same procedure. You may store the salve in a container for subsequent use.

Attention: In certain instances, chickweed can cause allergic skin responses. There have been reports of cattle dying after ingesting an excessive amount of the herb since the plant frequently releases saponins that are harmful at large concentrations. Although it would only take a few pounds to put the animal to death.

Cinnamon

Another well-known spice in the kitchen is cinnamon sticks. Cinnamon is also taken into account for its therapeutic properties. Even if it wasn't technically an herb, I still think it's important to include it in our list of plants and their applications. Typically, laurel family trees' inner bark is where cinnamon is found. It has been in use for a long time and was a popular item for trade in the past. Cinnamon was really 15 times more expensive in Rome in the first century A.D. than platinum. Cinnamon was most likely initially utilized as a medicinal plant by the Chinese, who employed it to treat fever and diarrhea. Modern research has demonstrated that cinnamon's insulin-like effects help diabetics control their blood sugar levels.

Medicinal Uses:

- Diabetes
- Mild Stimulant
- Aromatic Astringent
- Antimicrobial Relieves Gas

How to use ground cinnamon

Sri Lankan origin Taking 1 teaspoon of cinnamon powder daily to help lower blood sugar levels is the most important way to utilize cinnamon to treat diabetes. Cinnamon capsules can come in a variety of dosages, but in general, taking 1-6 grams of cinnamon capsules throughout the day is a good idea. A freshly ground cinnamon stick and 6 tablespoons of stevia are a nice little substitute for cinnamon sugar. This works well as a topping on toast, oatmeal, or fruit.

Although ground cinnamon is quite harmless, skin rashes can be caused by volatile oils. Small levels of coumarin are present in cassia and other cinnamons; typically, only excessive dosages of this molecule cause blood thinning and liver issues, but it is still important to be aware of this. Additionally, due to cinnamon's blood-thinning properties, you should cease using it at least one week before your operation. To prevent a hazardous reduction in blood pressure, you should be cautious about monitoring your blood sugar.

Clove

Simply put, clove buds are flower buds that must be gathered at the appropriate time. Prior to blossoming, the buds may become a deep crimson color; this is the optimum time to harvest your clove. An evergreen shrub with vivid pink flowers and violet berries sprouts clove buds. Planting cloves in warm, humid climates is the best course of action.

Clove's usage as a medicinal plant was first documented in history during the Han Dynasty in China, which lasted from 300 B.C. to 200 B.C. It was a priceless spice that once rivaled the value of oil, similar to cinnamon and clove. Next, let's investigate more closely to determine some of clove's key therapeutic benefits or potential applications.

Medicinal Uses :

- Analgesic
- Stimulant
- Antiseptic
- Anti-emetic
- Antoxidant
- Antimicrobial

How to use Clove Oil

Cloves or a few drops of clove oil applied to a cotton ball will relieve toothaches. However, you should exercise caution and avoid putting the oil directly on the gum while using this method.

To treat illnesses like shingles that cause nerve discomfort, distilled oil up to a maximum of 3 percent may be used topically. Clove powder can be used sparingly to relieve conditions including nausea, indigestion, and bloating.

Never take essential oils without first carefully diluting them, since this might lead to dermatitis in rare situations. Use clove carefully and pay attention to how your body responds to it.

Comfrey herbal

Comfrey has been used for centuries, at least since the time of the ancient Greeks. During the Middle Ages, the plant Confey was extensively grown in monastic gardens. Comfrey was a typical herb growing in many gardens across Europe and America in the 1700s and 1800s. However, research conducted somewhere in the late 1970s revealed that comfrey's internal usage can seriously harm the liver, leading to a tarnished reputation and even a ban on its use in several nations.

Products made from creams, poultices, or ointments are still regarded as safe. In certain western nations, as well as in Central Europe and the eastern United States, comfrey still grows wild.

Medicinal Uses:

- Anti-inflammatory
- Demulcent
- Wound healer
- Astringent

How to Use Comfrey Ointment

Today, using comfrey topically in gels, ointments, creams, liniments, or poultices is the most effective method. You may locate supplements that keep the pain-relieving and anti-inflammatory effects while swapping out toxic alkaloids. Any of these techniques should be used 3–4 times a day to treat a bruise, sore joint, or muscle.

Warning: As I already indicated, several nations have made it illegal to use Comfrey domestically; therefore, I must caution you one more time against doing so. The body's alkaloids can seriously harm the liver.

Dandelion

The dandelion is frequently seen as a weed since it can quickly cover a yard and suffocate vegetation. Dandelions entered our list of herbs since they are a lovely plant with a lot of health-related and nutritional advantages.

One of the nicest things about dandelion herb is that the entire plant—from the flower to the roots—can be used. The blooms can be consumed fresh, roasted, or converted into dandelion wine when they are still yellow. Salads taste amazing with the greens. The dandelion's core may even be ingested; it is typically roasted and eaten or used to make a delectable cup of tea.

A common nickname for dandelion is "piss-a-bed" due to its strong diuretic effects.

Medicinal Uses :

- Diuretic
- Liver Cleanser
- Strong laxative
- Kidney Cleanser

How to use Dandelion Tea

I already mentioned how the entire crop of dandelion may be utilized. The stomach, liver, and pancreas are just a few of the digestive organs where the root's therapeutic benefits are most evident.

The dandelion root has been demonstrated to have the capacity to balance blood sugar levels as well as promote digestive processes. The dandelion plant primarily benefits the lungs, aiding in water drainage and even weight reduction. Additionally, those who wish to decrease their blood pressure frequently use dandelion leaves. When combined with other herbs, it effectively treats skin issues like eczema, acne, and boils.

Attention: Dandelion is a healthy plant, but it might damage people who are allergic to ragweed. Additionally, confirm that the lions you select have not yet had a pesticide or herbicide spraying.

Echinacea

Echinacea, sometimes known as Black Sampson, is the plant right next to our collection of plants. Western original Americans used to call it snakeroot since it was once used to treat snake bites. The herb has also been utilized by locals to alleviate toothaches.

The two largest Indian tribes that utilized the herb were presumably the Omaha-Ponca and Cheyenne. As previously indicated, they used the liquids from the roots to cure toothaches as well as burns on their bodies. Echinacea is now utilized to boost the immune system and quicken the common cold's recovery.

Echinacea comes in three main varieties, with Echinacea purpurea being the most commonly used kind from Georgia to Texas, up to Michigan, and east to Ohio. People from regions like Michigan, Arkansas, Texas, and here in Nebraska can locate this species of Echinacea, which is most frequently seen in open woodlands and plains. Roadsides, prairies, and outcrops continue to be thriving habitats for Echinacea angustifolia, and residents in Texas may expect to see it growing as far north as Dakota and southern Saskatchewan, as well as in Montana and Colorado.

Medicinal Uses:

Colds and Fluss

Wound healer

Blood cleanser

Antibacterial

Antiviral Immune enhancement

To hasten the recovery from colds, chest infections, and sore throats, echinacea extract can be taken as a tincture, pill, or capsule. A tincture of echinacea that has been distilled can help reduce the symptoms of sore throats.

Simply chew the root of the echinacea plant to relieve toothaches. This method of treating a toothache is incredibly effective, and I can still remember using it in high school when we practiced scope evaluation. However, making the root into tea could be a better strategy than simply eating it.

Attention: Echinacea has occasionally been reported to produce an allergic response. This is most likely a result of the Asteraceae (Daisy) genus reacting. You shouldn't consume echinacea if you have an autoimmune disorder.

Garlic

Our list of herbs also includes another herb that is frequently used in cooking. The earliest Greek top athletes employed garlic, which has been used for hundreds of years and is believed to increase strength and endurance, making it one of the main quality-enhancing drugs. Garlic was also employed by witches and ghosts to fend off spells, curses, and charms. Garlic was created in the Middle Ages by the monasteries to heal intestinal, renal, and respiratory issues.

Many people claim that eating a lot of garlic during World War II helped the Russians survive in difficult circumstances. Garlic is now primarily used to treat and prevent heart disease, lower cholesterol, reduce high blood pressure, and strengthen the immune system. Wherever vegetable gardens can be established, garlic grows quite well.

Additionally, garlic can grow quite well indoors; all it takes is one garlic clove to produce a whole garlic plant. Take one of the garlic cloves you purchase the next time you go to the store and plant it pointed-end up in a specific area of wet soil. You'll soon have a healthy crop of garlic if you continue to water the clove every day. I want to include garlic in our list of herbs since it is one of the most vital and underutilized medicinal plants in the world.

Medicinal Uses:
- Antibiotic
- Reduces blood pressure

- Blood-thinner
- Provides helpful intestinal flora
- Counters cough and respiratory infection
- Antifungal
- Lowers cholesterol
- Diarrhea

How to use Garlic Capsules

Garlic that is organic is simply the finest kind to eat because cooking it destroys many of the compounds that give it its therapeutic benefits. In addition to eating fresh garlic, you can crush a few cloves with some olive oil and put them over a salad. Garlic pills are another option you have, and they're a terrific way to provide your body with the essential components of garlic. Try to seek out items that include allicin, one of the key components in garlic.

Warning: When used as part of a normal diet, garlic is generally healthy. There is a little possibility that consuming more than 4 cloves of garlic per day, which is the recommended daily intake, can harm the body's platelets, which prevent blood clots from forming. Garlic should be used at least two weeks before any kind of operation, especially if you take anticoagulant medication.

Ginger

Ginger is a popular herb from Asia that has been used in baking for more than 4,400 years. Indian, Chinese, and Arab remedies have employed it since antiquity. They believed it came from the Garden of Eden since it was so uncommon throughout the Middle Ages. You could learn today that ginger is used to cure motion sickness-related issues. The root is also used to make teas that are used to cure a variety of illnesses. At least 2,000 years ago, the Greeks and Romans were the ones who brought ginger to Europe for the first time. The Arabian Peninsula's trade was likely to blame for this.

Medicinal Uses:

- Fight infection
- Coughs and colds
- Morning sickness
- Nausea and vomiting
- Anti-emetic
- Anti-inflammatory

- Stimulates sweating
- Digestive tonic

How to use ginger root

Slice one inch of ginger root into small pieces, add two cups of water, and steep to produce a tasty ginger tea. Like many other herbs, ginger may also be found in capsule form. This is a fantastic method to receive your daily recommended amount of ginger. Although extracts can also be used, they are often exclusively employed in the diagnosis of osteoarthritis.

Although ginger is a relatively safe herb to take, it can occasionally induce heartburn. Pregnant women should likewise limit their daily intake to one gram. In actuality, you shouldn't use blood thinners with excessive amounts of ginger.

Ginkgo Biloba

For thousands of years, Ginkgo biloba has been employed in herbal therapy. Today, it is widely used in both the United States and Europe, with the Chinese perhaps having invented it first. Despite not being an herb you would grow in your yard, ginkgo truly originates from the leaf of the ginkgo tree, and I still believe it deserves a spot on our list of herbs.

Ginkgo biloba has earned a reputation for supporting the brain throughout time. Flavonoids and terpenoids, both of which are antioxidants, are the two main components of ginkgo, according to the University of Maryland Medical Center. Additionally, flavonoids have been demonstrated to support blood vessel, heart, and nerve protection. Terpenoids, which considerably increase blood circulation by dilating blood vessels and preventing platelets from adhering to one another, are likely the reason why ginkgo has a reputation for being good for the brain.

Medicinal Uses :

- Mental Health
- Antioxidant
- Boost circulation
- Protects nerve tissue

How to use Ginkgo capsules

As I just explained, ginkgo helps increase blood circulation, so it should come as no surprise that this herb will help with cognition and memory. It has previously been demonstrated to be effective in treating symptoms of the central nervous system, including vertigo and tinnitus. Ginkgo doesn't just improve circulation in the brain; it also improves circulation throughout the entire body, from the feet to the head. Ginkgo is normally taken orally in the form of capsules.

Warning: It is important to keep in mind that you should stop taking Ginkgo at least three days before surgery if you are taking medicine to prevent blood clots.

Lavender

The aroma of lavender fields is perhaps what makes them most famous, and it's the ideal plant to utilize on a busy day. Given its relaxing properties, lavender is frequently utilized in soaps, detergents, and essential oils. For the same purpose, lavender is frequently added to teas. Lavender has a roughly 2500-year history that begins in the Mediterranean. It is mostly grown nowadays for use in essential oils. Lavender has many other culinary uses besides making tea, and a little sugar may enhance the fragrant flavor. Some seafood, soups, salads, and baked products pair well with it.

Medicinal uses

- Antidepressant
- Sedation Symptoms
- Antiseptic
- Analgesic Relieves
- Gas Antispasmodic

How to Use Lavender Essential Oil

Lavender is extensively used for its essential oil, which has relaxing, soothing, and energizing properties that make it the best treatment for headaches. Put a few drops in your bathtub or add some to your homemade soap. I like to put a few drops from my humidifier in the pill bowl.

This is a fantastic technique to disperse lavender oil around your room and maintain a higher humidity level. You may also massage lavender oil into your skin to ease any pain you may be experiencing. Adding a few lavender sprigs to your cup of tea while it steeps will also allow the tea to benefit from the health benefits of lavender.

Although I wouldn't advise taking the essential oil directly, lavender is really a fairly safe plant to consume. However, doing so might have unintended adverse effects.

Lemon Balm

herb, lemon balm Another herb with a strong scent is lemon balm, which releases a scent of lemon and mint from its leaves. Lemon balm has been used in herbal therapy for a very long time, dating back to the Greeks more than 2000 years ago. Back then, to reduce fever, both the Greeks and the Romans would add lemon balm to their wine. To aid in relaxation and sleep, lemon balm is now frequently mixed with other herbs like valerian and hops.

Along with certain other nootropics, it is becoming more and more popular, and some studies have indicated that it also enhances memory and learning. So it should come as no surprise that several herbalists are recommending lemon balm for the treatment of Alzheimer's.

Medicinal uses:

- Insect repellent
- Antispasmodic
- Relieves Gas
- Relaxant
- Antiviral
- Antidepressant Depression and Pressure

How to Use Lemon Balm Tea

Lemon balm may be used in a wide variety of ways, making it a flexible plant in terms of the ailments it treats and the manner in which it can be used. Use lemon balm to its fullest potential in teas. A cup of water should be steeped with five to six fresh leaves for six minutes under pressure. To sweeten the deal, think about adding some honey or stevia. You can also add some mint to provide a little more heat. Ointments, tinctures, and aggregates are all readily accessible and quite effective treatments for lemon balm.

Neem

Neem has a very long history of use as a remedy; in fact, neem may be found in one of the world's oldest writings. Neem's medicinal benefits are mentioned in several classical Sanskrit texts, and the Sanskrit term for neem, nimba, really means "good health." Neem is a tree; therefore, it would be challenging for some people to classify it as an herb, but I had to include it in our list of herbs anyway. Neem should be acknowledged while discussing herbs because it has been used by the Indians for more than 4,000 years. Neem is now employed for a number of purposes, including the treatment of psoriasis, eczema, scabies, and other skin conditions. Neem is well known for its health advantages for your body in addition to its benefits for your skin.

Medicinal Uses:

- Blood Moisturizer
- Lowers blood sugar rates
- Anitbacterial
- Antifungal
- Relieves itchyness
- Anti-inflammatory Immune help

How to use neem

Neem may be used as a skin toner by simply boiling 20 of the leaves in half a liter of water. Once the leaves have become mushy and discolored and the liquid has turned green, they should be strained. Hold the water in the glass and, when you're ready to use it, put the cotton ball that has been saturated with the liquid on your head. By doing this, acne and blackheads won't appear. You may use it to prevent skin diseases by simply filling your tub with a lot of water.

Neem may currently only be administered to youngsters, so use caution. Neem should not be taken by pregnant or breastfeeding women.

Nettle Stinging

In Nebraska, stinging nettles should be a prolific plant. They are interesting herbs. The most well-known characteristic of stinging nettles is their It was their sting, as you suspected. The nettle plant possesses sharp spines that emerge upon touch and unleash a cocktail of chemicals into the bloodstream as soon as they absorb the victim's skin.

As a result of the nettle plant's production of histamine, acetylcholine, dopamine, and formic acid, you get the burning or biting sensation. Surprisingly, the plant itself may be used to treat the burning feeling;

the afflicted region can be treated with nettle leaf juice. Nettle leaf has a severe sting, but other than that, it is a truly beneficial plant that warrants a spot on our list of herbs.

Medicinal Uses:

- Anti-allergenic
- Diuretic
- Anti-inflammatory
- Blood Cleanser Tonic

When to use Nettle Leaf

The nettle plant may be taken in many different ways; nettle teas, capsules, tinctures, and extracts are all excellent methods to reap its benefits. To effectively treat hay fever symptoms, capsules are available; 300 to 800 mg are typically recommended. Because of the potent diuretic effects that nettles have, they are frequently used in teas to treat conditions including diabetes, prostate health, and high blood pressure.

Nettles may have a few negative effects that you should be aware of. Impotence, redness, and an upset stomach are all possible, although they are uncommon. Before consuming nettle, you should see your doctor if you are taking medication for diabetes, high blood pressure, anxiety, or sleeplessness.

Oregano

Oregano plant Another herb used in cooking frequently appears on our list of healing plants. As far as culinary herbs go, oregano is listed. I enjoy this material. Clearly a member of the mint family, oregano originated in the warm regions of Eurasia and the Mediterranean. Oregano was initially utilized by the Greeks in antiquity, who said that the goddess Aphrodite created it. Oregano is derived from two Greek words: oros, which means "mountain," and ganos, which means "joy." When you combine the two words, you get "joy of the mountains." Oregano didn't truly become popular as a medical herb until the Middle Ages, when people started using it to cure coughs, indigestion, toothaches, and rheumatism.

Medicinal Uses:

- Antifungal
- Expectorant Stimulant
- Antiseptic
- Antioxidant

How to use oregano Oil

There are many uses for oregano in the kitchen, as you might have already guessed. These are all excellent methods since oregano may be used for purposes other than seasoning pasta dishes. It is the ideal technique to hasten the healing of an illness. Make tea out of it. Ringworm, sports foot, and warts may all be treated topically using oregano oil that has been distilled in coconut or olive oil.

Warning: While oregano is fantastic for many individuals, some people will discover that the oil irritates their skin. Because of this, just a tiny quantity should be used to test the water, and when using it, be sure you only use distilled oregano oil.

Peppermint

Because of the lovely perfume that the damaged leaves of the peppermint plant may produce, it is so widely recognized today. It's difficult to leave peppermint off our list of herbs because it's utilized in so many different ways, both culinary and medicinal. Since peppermint is a cross between spearmint and water mint, it truly originated in England sometime in the late seventeenth century. Additionally popular in ancient Egypt, where it was used to treat indigestion, dried peppermint leaves have even been discovered inside the pyramids that the Egyptians constructed. In Western Europe throughout the 18th century, peppermint was widely used to cure respiratory infections, morning sickness, and diarrhea.

Principal Medical Uses: alleviates gas Very acidic, powerful sedative Antiseptic Diaphoretic, a mild analgesic Antispasmodic.

How to Use Peppermint Oil Peppermint

The herb peppermint is great for treating fevers and colds. Due to the presence of menthol inside the peppermint plant, peppermint has the ability to reduce the discomfort associated with sore throats. It's a terrific approach to lessening the effects of a sore throat to make a tea with some peppermint and some lemon sugar. Consider adding some peppermint oil to your humidifier (those with the medication chamber) if you have sinus congestion.

Warning: Although peppermint is a highly beneficial plant to use, if you have sensitive skin, you may want to avoid its oil or dilute it to prevent irritation.

Plantain Leaves

One of the earliest plants to go from Europe to America was possibly plantain. Because of his capacity to flourish anywhere the contemporary conquerors had ever put it, the indigenous people gave him the nickname "white man's footprint" after the Puritan plantain colonists who first brought him over. Plantain grows all throughout the world and is currently frequently seen as a weed, yet it has some potent therapeutic properties that should not be overlooked. Plantains' ability to treat injuries including burns, edema, and bruising has been documented since medieval Europe. Plantain has demonstrated excellent results in the treatment of illnesses including edema, jaundice, ear infections, ringworm, and shingles, in addition to being a potent wound healer. The key ingredients that give plantains their medicinal benefits include aucubin, allatonine, mucilage, flavonoids, caffeic acid, and alcohols that are found in the wax of plantain leaves. It is essential to include it in your natural first aid kit because of all of these factors.

Medicinal Uses:

- Wound healer
- Anticatarrhal
- Anti-inflammatory
- Analgesic Antiviral

How to use plantain leaves

By applying salve or tincture to the affected region, plantains can be used to cure depression. Crushing the leaves also works well as sunburn therapy. You can see that plantains make excellent herbs for any prepper just from these two uses, but the benefits of plantains don't end there. Plantain is a fantastic herb to know when in the woods and keep in your herbal first aid box since it can classify cuts and mend wounds. By making tea with it, plantains may also be used to combat infections, colds, and flu.

Sage Plant

Like the majority of culinary herbs, sage also has some therapeutic qualities. It features applications that make it simpler to deal with colds, coughs, and sore throats. In the past, sage was used in Egypt to fend off evil, heal snakebite wounds, and increase female fertility. Sage was also used in India to treat heartburn and sore throats. Since the Middle Ages, when the Romans introduced sage to Europe, it has been grown in herb gardens and kitchens. Sage is a common ingredient in many natural products on the market today. Sage is a great herb for survivalists since it allows them to create these organic items. Sage is frequently used to make deodorants because of its antiperspirant properties, and mouthwash is widely used because of the sage's ability to destroy microorganisms.

How to Use Organic Salvian Tee

The benefits of sage can be obtained through tea. It just takes 10 minutes to soak 1 tablespoon of sage in 1 cup of water. By mixing sage and thyme, you may also create a fairly amazing sore throat remedy. Add 16 ounces of apple cider vinegar to one ounce of each of them. Before using, give it 10 days to relax and give it regular shakes.

Caution: Sage, however, should be used with caution as it includes substances called thujones in its essential oils. In typical culinary uses, it is nutritious, but greater amounts should be used with caution, and alcohol extracts are not recommended.

Skullcap

The original therapeutic usage of skullcap, a plant in the mint family, was often discovered through researching the lives of the native Americans. The roots of skullcap have been utilized as a treatment for renal and gastrointestinal issues. Skullcap didn't establish its reputation as a sedative until the settlers came. They utilized it to treat a wide range of conditions, including illness, nervousness, and even rabies.

Skullcap is most frequently used as a benign pain reliever to treat fibromyalgia, tension headaches, anxiety, and insomnia. You must be aware of the Chinese variety as well as the North American range while cultivating skull caps for your herb garden.

The Chinese skullcap is a far more resilient type that thrives in both warm and chilly areas and does exceptionally well during droughts. The circumstances, however, must be more precise for the North American type to flourish since it needs a highly rich, wet, and somewhat acidic soil.

Main Medicinal use:

- Sedative
- Strong bitter Nerve tonic
- Antispasmodic

How to use skullcap capsules

One ounce of skullcap can be fermented in a pint of boiling water for around ten minutes to make skullcap tea. Drink this every several hours in amounts of 1/2 cup to ease headaches and anxiety. If you don't have time to prepare a cup of tea, capsules are also a fantastic and efficient way to enjoy the benefits of skullcap.

Skullcap is a powerful medicine that should be taken with caution since some studies indicate that it might cause liver damage. If you have liver problems, you should only use a skullcap.

Turmeric

Although turmeric is more of a spice than an herb, I had to include it on the list of herbs. Hinduism has a long history with turmeric, which is associated with fertility and purity. Even today, Hindu brides still take part in a custom that involves applying turmeric paste to their faces before saying their vows. Turmeric was formerly referred to by Marco Polo as a vegetable having saffron-like qualities. Westerners didn't start to appreciate turmeric's therapeutic properties until about the middle of the 20th century.

Turmeric's major therapeutic component, curcumin, has an approximate 3-percent curcumin content; for this reason, it is more advantageous to consume a turmeric extract.

How to Use Turmeric Powder

Eating turmeric is one of the best and most well-known ways to reap its advantages. Although it may not be simple, adding it to meals is a fantastic method. Don't be misled into believing that the only way to enjoy the health benefits of this lovely herb is to consume it in cuisine. You can also add it to drinks or use it as toothpaste by dipping your toothbrush in some turmeric powder and brushing your teeth for around three minutes. Your teeth won't get stained, but your toothbrush or sink won't be immune. Turmeric powder can also be combined with a little water to create a paste that can be applied topically.

Valerian

Valerian root has to be my personal favorite so far for promoting calm. The Greeks and Romans undoubtedly utilized valerian for the first time in history, along with many other plants on this list. Disorders of the digestive system, urinary tract, and liver were all treated with valerian.

In the past, valerian was utilized to treat those who had the condition. Valerian will be entertaining, even for the cat! In the same manner that we use catnip now, people still use valerian. Many individuals believed that the cat's response to the herb might be used to gauge the potency of valerian. Rats that emit an offensive odor are cat attractants and have been known to be caught in rat traps in the past. Today, valerian root is most frequently used as a supplement for promoting sleep and reducing anxiety.

How to use Valerian root capsules

Here's what I do to get a better night's sleep: I take 2-3 Valerian root capsules together with 5 mg of melatonin, and it works extremely well to give me a restful night's sleep. It doesn't really overpower me, but sitting there all night helps put me in a sleep state.

Although valerian is usually considered to be relatively safe, there are some potential adverse effects that you should be aware of. You may want to discontinue using it if you have a headache, nausea, or upper stomach pain. Sleepiness, dry mouth, odd nightmares, and brain fog are among the less severe side effects.

Witch Hazel

Though I've just recently learned, native Americans have long employed the peculiar herb known as witch hazel. Witch hazel was utilized as a magic tool to locate untapped supplies of water and/or priceless minerals when I was researching it. I had mistakenly believed that Witch Hazel had some sort of reputation for fending against witches. Although some people may not consider witch hazel to be a weed because it is a woody shrub, I had to include it in the category of herbs along with its applications because of its excellent astringent and antibacterial properties. Nowadays, you can get witch hazel liquid (an alcohol extract from twigs) in practically every pharmacy store. The sample often contains very little active drug; therefore, the majority of symptoms will really be caused by the alcohol itself. This is the sole downside.

How to use witch hazel tonic

Making a tonic using witch hazel is the best use for it. For this, you'll need vodka, distilled water, and 1/2 lb. witch hazel tree bark. Witch hazel should be combined with water to cover the bark by one to two inches. For about 20 minutes, boil, then cover and simmer. After filtering off the bark, add half of the tea's volume to the alcohol. Therefore, add 10 ounces of alcohol to 20 ounces of tea. If you just want the toner pre-made to include additional aloe vera, Thayer's is a great option.

Yarrow plant

The herb yarrow is ideal for all-natural first-aid kits. It works well to halt the blood flow from small cuts, mend bruises, and treat cold, flu, and fever-related symptoms. Native Americans gave this "living medication" the name "Yarrow" and used it to treat both toothaches and earaches. Although it is rumored that the Greek hero Achilles employed yarrow to heal his soldiers during the Trojan War, the genus Achillea of yarrow really gets its name from Achilles. Yarrow has been utilized as a backup herb by several individuals throughout human history, which is why I decided to add it to our list of herbs.

Principal Medical Uses Astringent Intestinal tonic increases blood vessel strength and reduces hemorrhage. Healer of wounds induces vomiting and lowers fever.

How to use Yarrow Tea

Drinking yarrow as a tea is a terrific way to experience its benefits; this may be done to reduce fatigue and hasten the recovery from colds and the flu. Additionally, yarrow may be made into a cream or ointment that can be applied to tiny injuries to reduce or stop bleeding.

Use yarrow with caution if you are pregnant or breastfeeding since it has been found to cause allergic reactions in very rare circumstances, especially when applied to the body.

Anthemis nobilis chamomile It is believed that chamomile might reduce fatigue and gastrointestinal discomfort or inflammation. Joint cramps are only one of the numerous aches and pains that the floral oil may treat. Managing menstrual cycles and recovering from headaches are two other benefits of chamomile.

Cinquefoil

To lessen inflammation, apply cinnamon. Ulcers and swollen mouths may also be treated with it. Jaundice is known to be treated with the juice. Cinquefoil may be used to treat sore joints in addition to helping to hoarse the throat and cough.

Columbine

Aquilegia vulgaris (Columbine) is a somewhat poisonous plant; hence, its astringent components are mostly used topically and as lotions.

Feverfew
Fever and migraine headaches can both be effectively treated with feverfew. It could also aid in the relief of ailments like arthritis.

Foxglove Digitalis purpurea
The pure variety of the crop is employed to enhance cardiac contractility and regulate heart rhythm.

Golden Rod
The golden rod can be used to treat eczema, arthritis, and painful menstruation. To aid in the healing of skin ulcers, it can be applied externally.

Lady's Mantle-Lchemilla
This spice has been used to treat too heavy periods. Stopping the bleeding at the lady's mantle's root has been advised.

Lavender
Lavender reduces nausea and prevents dizziness. It is frequently included in therapeutic baths as an oil to ease tension. Also, it could reduce blood pressure. Skin conditions, including eczema and psoriasis, can be treated with a modest dose.

Lovage
As a digestive aid, lovage is utilized. This lessens the pain from inside. It is also known that this plant might lessen eye redness.

Pennyroyal
Headaches are believed to be relieved by pennyroyal. It has been used to alleviate the stomach pain associated with colic. Additionally, it has a reputation for reducing feverish whooping cough and measles symptoms.

Poppy–Papaver Rhoeas
Poppy is used to relieve coughs and make people feel worn out. Whooping cough, angina, asthma, and bronchitis may all be treated with petals.

Primrose–Primula vulgaris

Sedative primrose encourages rest and sleep by lowering tension. Taken in spoonfuls, root infusion is effective in the management of headaches. In addition, it has been used to treat rheumatism and gout.

Rosemary-Rosmarinus

Rosemary has been used to treat asthma, poor circulation, and nausea. Additionally, it may be used to cure fever and as a mouthwash to clean surfaces. Additionally, it is said to reduce dandruff and enhance memory.

Sage–Salvia

Hoarseness, coughing, and headaches can all be treated with sage. One of the best-known treatments for tonsillitis, laryngitis, and sore throats The plant's honey-sweetened infusion encourages menstruation and has a mild laxative effect.

Sorrel–Rumex acetosella

Sorrel leaves are known for quenching thirst and reducing fever. These leaves also have diuretic properties.

Vervain–Verbena officinalis

Vervain is regarded as an effective remedy for colds and coughs. It alleviates the wheezing and breathlessness that accompany fever.

Wintergreen–Pyrola minor

The calming properties of wintergreen are well known, and they flavor everything from gum to mouthwash. In medicine, it can be used locally on wounds and taken orally to treat bladder and kidney ulcers. An organic antimicrobial is present in the plant.

Woodruffe

Since woodruff has relaxing properties, it can be used to treat insomnia. It can strengthen the abdomen and clear colon blockages when administered as an injection.

Yarrow Achillea millefolium

For skin blemishes, wounds, and abrasions, yarrow is used topically. It is known that yarrow infusions might hasten the healing process after really bad bruises. Hay fever is one of the allergic mucous issues for which yarrow flowers are utilized.

PART 6

HERBAL TREATMENT FOR ANXIETY

Numerous herbal medicines have been studied as potential anti-anxiety treatments, but more research is required to fully grasp the dangers and advantages. Here's what we believe, Kava, and you don't know it. Although evidence of severe liver damage, including from short-term use, led the Food and Drug Administration to issue cautions regarding the use of kava-containing nutritional supplements, kava has been shown to be a possible treatment for depression. Even if the early allegations of liver damage have been refuted, if you're thinking about taking kava-containing goods, proceed with additional caution and see your doctor.

The love rose. The results of a few small clinical investigations suggest that passion flowers may reduce anxiety. It might be challenging to distinguish between the distinctive properties of each plant because passion flowers are frequently blended with other herbs in commercial goods. When used as directed, passion flower is often regarded as healthful, although some studies have discovered that it can make people feel sleepy, lightheaded, and indecisive.

Valerian. According to certain studies, valerian users reported less worry and tension. People in other studies said there was no advantage. At approved doses, valerian is often regarded as safe, but because there aren't any studies on its long-term safety, you shouldn't take it for longer than a few weeks at a time without your doctor's approval. It may cause adverse reactions, including headaches, wooziness, and somnolence.

Chamomile. According to research, using chamomile for a brief period of time is usually regarded as healthy and can assist with anxiety symptoms. However, chamomile may make bleeding more likely if used with blood-thinning medication. Some people who are sensitive to plants in the Chamaemilia family, including chamomile, may experience allergic reactions when exposed to chamomile. Ragweed, marigolds, daisies, and chrysanthemums are other members of the same family.

Hey, lavender. There is some preliminary and limited evidence that taking oral lavender or using lavender aromatherapy helps relieve stress. Additionally, it could make you hungry, enhance the calming effects of other drugs and foods, and lower your blood pressure.

Lemon balm, that is. According to a preliminary study, lemon balm can lessen some anxiety feelings, including trepidation and anticipation. Lemon balm is often well absorbed and regarded as safe for short-term use; however, it might cause nausea and discomfort in the abdomen. Lemon balm is an extract that is often sold in capsule form. It can be consumed alone or combined with herbal tea. Since at least the Middle Ages, people have used this common anxiety treatment to ease symptoms and promote calm. Additionally, lemon balm may be helpful for treating headaches and gastrointestinal issues. Numerous studies have revealed that lemon balm, which is well-known for its calming and sedative effects, may also improve mood and lessen stress in addition to easing anxiety.

Anxiety may wreak havoc on your daily life and general well-being. Finding a workable solution to handle your symptoms is crucial to reducing them. The body's natural reaction to anything unfamiliar or intimidating is anxiety. It's not intended to have the ability to control your life, though.

Keep in mind that because every person is unique, there might be variations in how the body responds to natural therapies. Herbal remedies help us relax. They're an ideal approach to safely and effectively controlling and treating anxiety symptoms.

In contrast to how medicines are utilized, herbal remedies are not subject to FDA regulation. The quality of some pharmaceuticals may still be an issue despite the strengthened quality control measures in place since 2010. Keep in mind that nature is not necessarily safe.

Consult your doctor before using any herbal supplements to treat your anxiety, especially if you already take other medications. Some natural treatments and some pharmaceuticals may interact with severe adverse effects.

Many herbal pills used to treat depression may make you feel tired, making them potentially unsafe to consume while operating machinery or performing other risky duties. If you decide to use herbal supplements, your doctor may be able to help you understand the possible dangers and advantages.

If your anxiety affects your daily activities, talk to your doctor. In order to improve symptoms, more severe kinds of anxiety typically need medical care or psychological counseling (psychotherapy).

PART 7

MEDICINAL HERBS TO BOOST THE IMMUNE SYSTEM

The list of herbs that may be used to strengthen one's immune system is provided below:

Black Elderberry

It is a fantastic herb that aids in enhancing tissue oxygenation and circulation to provide the body with the nutrients required to ward off sickness. Elderberry, often known as a relaxant, is a great remedy for croup and vomiting in boys since it helps to reduce spasmodic cough. Flavonoids, which have antibacterial effects within the body and help reinforce cell membranes to prevent viruses from hanging around, are abundant in berries and flowers.

Peppermint

The leaf contains potassium, magnesium, B vitamins, vitamin C, and other nutrients that support a healthy immune system. Because of its paradoxically cool flavor and its calming and relaxing after-effects on the skin, peppermint is frequently used as a cure for fever and chills, which can be partially explained by these factors.

This tea is helpful for the flu since it also fights germs and helps relax the digestive tract.

Thyme leaf

Thyme is native to the Mediterranean Sea, but it thrives well here and is now a common addition to any neighborhood herb garden. Tea made from thyme leaves is a delicious cough suppressant. Excess mucus is forced out of the lungs, which helps to calm irritated lung tissue. Thyme's volatile oils, which have the tendency to open pores and thin phlegm, give it a significant detoxifying and penetrating action.

It is a common active treatment for strong infectious species like typhoid and diphtheria, and it is also known to be antibacterial and anti-inflammatory to the lungs. Thyme is now used to treat postnasal drip, whooping cough, sore throats, persistent colds, and bronchitis.

Sage plant

It grows nicely in herb gardens and is a native of the Mediterranean. The ideal sore throat cure is sage leaf tea. It helps break up the formation of mucus and has a special impact on relieving throat irritation. Additionally, it contains thujone, a potent antiseptic and antibiotic that guards against dangerous infections, germs, and fungus to hasten the body's immune system's recovery.

Osha root

Osha often thrives at high altitudes close to rocky rocks and cascades; however, the Ligusticum scoticum plant, a less aggressive relative, may be found in BC woodlands. The root's resins remove mucus from the lungs and sinuses to ease congestion. They also reduce inflammation by boosting your body's natural cortisol production. Osha is frequently used for colds, bronchitis, sinusitis, pneumonia, and the flu. Osha must be suspended throughout labor and delivery.

Ginger

During the cold and flu seasons, ginger is wonderful for improving your general immunity in addition to soothing your stomach.

Simply add the ginger and then link it to the milk, juice, or both. Simply add the ginger and then link it to the milk, juice, or both.

This adaptable herb's natural flame adds to many various applications and is antibacterial, antibiotic, and anti-inflammatory. Drink ginger tea, visit the juice bar for a fresh ginger shot if you're feeling crummy, or add more ginger to your cuisine.

Although it is generally safe when used in recipes and treatments, pregnant women shouldn't consume more than 2 grams of dried ginger each day.

The properties of Garlic

Garlic is much more than just a flavor enhancer. Although the research is still preliminary, it is thought to boost white blood cell performance and stimulate the immune system.

Enjoy garlic every day to keep you looking great because it's so easy to use. When you're ill, increase your consumption of garlic as well. Make a delicious garlic soup (don't skimp on the bone broth, though), eat some whole garlic cloves, roast a garlic bulb, or put some garlic in a jar of honey and let it sit for a few weeks to infuse.

Garlic in dietary amounts is relatively harmless. Although it would be impossible to consume enough to harm you, use caution if you use anti-clotting drugs. (And make sure to brush your teeth if you see yourself getting high on raw garlic, too!) Cinder Fire The best cooking medicine is this potent beverage, also known as Master Tonic, which is made from a potent mixture of apple cider vinegar, garlic, ginger, onion, horseradish, and hot peppers (plus a variety of other immune-boosting ingredients like turmeric or delicious ones like lemon or rosemary).

The combined strength of these sinus-clearing, warming, and infectious-fighting herbs, together with a boost from fermented vinegar, is what gives fire cider its efficacy. And yes, this drink will burn (in a good way!) as it is consumed.

Bitters can help your immune system by increasing it. Astragalus root, ginger, angelica root, and honey are the main constituents in this nourishing tonic; all of them have been shown to support immune system function.

An important plant in Chinese medicine known as astragalus has anti-inflammatory and antibacterial effects. According to an astragalus study, the root can boost infection resistance and control the immune system of the body.

Angelica root has also been demonstrated to alter the immune system and ease cold and respiratory symptoms.

Last but not least, ginger and honey are strong antioxidants with anti-bacterial and anti-inflammatory properties.

Honey inhibits cell growth and causes the immune system to respond to infection. Similar to turmeric, ginger contains anti-inflammatory properties and may ease muscular pain.

Recipe for immunosuppressive bitters

Contains 1 teaspoon. 1 ounce each of sweetie and dry astragalus root. 1/2 oz. of dried angelica root dried chamomile, 1 teaspoon. Dry ginger, 1 teaspoon. 1-stick of cinnamon a teaspoon of dried orange peel. Cardamom seed, 10 oz. (We propose vodka at 100 proof.) Direction In two tablespoons of hot water, dissolve the honey.

Method:

Apply the liquor to the jar's rim before adding the honey and the following seven components:

- Put the bitters in a cool, dark area and firmly seal them.
- If you want the bitters to be a certain strength, let them steep for around 2-4 weeks. Regularly (approximately once per day), shake the jars.
- When ready, strain the bitters through a coffee filter or muslin cheese cloth. At room temperature, put the soaked bitters in an airtight container.

For safety throughout the cold and flu season, mix this tonic with hot tea or take a few drops as though you were the first person to wake up.

PART 8

MEDICINAL HERBS TO LOSE WEIGHT

You're probably considering starting a diet if you're starting to feel self-conscious about your body mass since you're having problems attempting to fit into a swimsuit or clothing. The good news is that there are many terrific programs that may help you, many of which take a conventional approach and include using plants as a weight reduction system as one of their methods.

The many methods by which herbs can be utilized to aid in weight loss, reduce appetite, and curb food cravings are listed below. Boost the body's ability to burn fat more quickly and its metabolism.

improves the digestive system's capacity to break down food more rapidly and effectively. helps the body produce more blood sugar by carefully regulating how carbs and sugar are processed. increases the liver's ability to function more effectively.

One of the newest, most potent, and healthiest herbal weight loss solutions is green tea. This plant causes the skin to oxidize fuel, which can increase calorie burning. It also has a lot of antioxidants, which are beneficial for your heart and can boost your vitality. It is simple to obtain green tea, which may be used as a tea beverage or as a nutritional tablet supplement. This is one of the greatest herbs for weight loss, regardless of how you try to take it.

Dandelion: This plant is already well-known for improving digestion and has the potential to act as a mild laxative. Although it comes as a tablet, most people consume it uncooked by adding it to a vegetable salad.

Though less well-known than other natural substances, garcinia cambogia has been shown to be quite efficient in boosting the body's metabolic rate and acting as an appetite suppressor. This plant is frequently combined with other herbal substances when used in potent diet tablets.

Hoodia: This traditional plant is used to control hunger and food cravings. Usually, when someone consumes less, their body is depleted of food and gets more energy from burning fat more quickly.

L-methionine: This drug ingredient works with the liver to increase fat burning.

Seaweed, often known as kelp, is a known thyroid stimulant that also speeds up the body's metabolism and ability to burn fat. It can be consumed in its purest form or as an alternative to tablets.

The herb Cascara sagrada is used with colon-cleansing diets to eliminate waste and impurities from the skin. The plant is a strong laxative, and it is recommended that you use it for no longer than one week at a time to prevent potential adverse effects, including exhaustion and famine.

Cayenne: This plant is frequently used in recipes that are spicy. Capsaicin, a component in cayenne, has been demonstrated to support the body's ability to digest food and speed up metabolism, facilitating faster fat burning.

Ginseng: This traditional Chinese herb is renowned for its capacity to raise energy levels while also speeding up the body's metabolic rate.

Threatening Plants There may be negative side effects from using many plants in dietary supplements. One of these weeds is ephedra. Ephedra may still be found in a number of dietary supplements and has been demonstrated to be effective in assisting others in losing weight. However, this plant should be avoided since it has been linked to harmful side effects including hypertension, palpitations, and an accelerated heart rate.

Although dietary modifications combined with the use of herbs for weight loss are quite effective, they shouldn't be the only method of calorie burning and weight loss. Positive long-term weight reduction is more likely to be successful when combined with nutrition and exercise, such as leading a healthy lifestyle and engaging in regular exercise. Exercise at least three days a week, together with a reduction in calorie intake and sugar consumption, has been touted as one of the greatest strategies to consistently lose weightg-term weight reduction is more likely to be successful when combined with nutrition and exercise, such as leading a healthy lifestyle and engaging in regular exercise. Exercise at least three days a week, together with a reduction in calorie intake and sugar consumption, has been touted as one of the greatest strategies to consistently lose weight. Utilizing weight loss tablets in addition to these lifestyle adjustments will significantly increase your capacity to keep extra weight off and help you reach your ideal weight.

PART 9

MEDICINAL HERBS TO CURE INSOMNIA

A feeling of relaxation and renewal is the first result of getting a good night's sleep. Anyone who has gone more than one night without enough sleep can attest to this. The problems are just getting worse for those who are still alive after a week. Impaired attention, anger, and slower reaction times are all signs of insufficient sleep. You can see how harmful a lack of sleep may be by imagining yourself exhibiting all of these symptoms while operating a vehicle.

Sleep difficulties may worsen and have a detrimental impact on your health if they persist for an extended period of time. You could have cardiac issues as a result of certain sleep issues, or you might just feel so exhausted during the day that you are unable to work. Lack of sleep may do much more than just make you exhausted, despite what you might believe. For instance, the cause of your sleep issues will determine whether specific health issues develop, but a persistent lack of sleep might have no beneficial effects. In most circumstances, taking herbs for sleep can help ease these issues.

If you don't get enough good, restful sleep, you can eat well and exercise often and still be in bad health. A person's cognitive function and judgment, motor skills and reflexes, behavior, and mental health can all suffer adversely from even one night of inadequate sleep or sleep deprivation.

With all of this in mind, it is alarming to learn that about 30% of the general population has sleep problems and bad sleeping habits. 30% of the population cannot function at their highest level or enjoy life to the fullest.

Stress and worry are only two of the numerous things that might interfere with sleep. Whether going through a significant transition in their lives or having a severe issue at work or in their personal lives, the majority of individuals will find themselves tossing and turning in bed and unable to fall asleep. It is always better to speak with your doctor if the situation is serious, such as with persistent insomnia. We can suggest lifestyle adjustments, a prescription sleep aid, or a referral to a sleep expert.

If you fly and occasionally have jet lag or if you discover that your sleep issues are not severe enough to require a doctor's visit, you may want to investigate a homeopathic sleep remedy, including herbs. These are a few natural sleep aids and herbal cures that might assist you in getting a good night's rest.

One of the most commonly utilized calming herbs is lavender. It has been demonstrated to be useful in calming tense muscles and promoting sleep in certain people. Additionally, lavender has been shown to improve the quality of your sleep, enabling you to sleep through the night.

Essential oils are likely the most popular form of it. Spraying lavender oil in your bedroom 30 minutes before bed is a terrific idea. Additionally, lavender tea is particularly well-liked. It is a popular component in fragrances and bath and body products because of its alluring aroma. It has been shown that some people with mixed anxiety disorders might sleep better after using lavender oil as a treatment.

Chamomile: Chamomile is one of the most well-known plants for aiding sleep. Chamomile tea comes to mind when someone is looking for a natural solution for sadness or anxiety or if they are having problems falling asleep. The herb chamomile is frequently used as a mild sedative and may even assist in treating cardiac conditions and boosting the immune system.

The majority of herbal infusions and herbal medications contain this daisy-like shrub. In fact, if they don't want to use medications or other sleep aids, most individuals resort to herbal teas as a quick fix for insomnia. Take camomile tea at night as part of a regular self-care regimen to make it even easier. In addition to chamomile, relaxing activities like a warm bath or meditation can help encourage a sound sleep cycle and enhance the quality of sleep.

If you're looking for a pill-shaped sleep aid but don't want to use sedatives or even melatonin, try magnolia bark. Users should often start with the lowest dose, as advised. Magnolia is one of the plants that promotes sleep the most effectively, making it unwise to consume it during the day or while operating a motor vehicle. It is believed to function by relaxing the mind, resulting in somnolence and deep REM sleep.

Short-term, one capsule per day should be sufficient to change your skin's circadian cycle. The herb magnolia bark also has the benefit of lowering cortisol levels in the body, which is a stress hormone, when taken orally.

While magnolia bark exhibits favorable sleep benefits, it is vital to understand that, as with many active botanicals, medication interactions must be taken into consideration. Before attempting to use herbal supplements like magnolia bark, please check with your doctor if you are already on any other drugs.

Virlian Root The root is utilized for medical purposes, while the plant is well-known for its alluring scent and is used in fragrances, bath products, and body care products. While valer root may not make you as drowsy as other sleeping herbs, it is known to promote relaxation. Sleeping herbs come in a variety of potencies. Although there is still some additional work to be done, Valerian can assist in calming your racing thoughts at night so that you can sleep better. One of the numerous plants that have been used for centuries and go all the way back to the Greek and Roman eras is valerian root.

As previously said, it is quite mild, and while it is frequently consumed in the form of tea, it is also available in the form of capsules, nutritional tablets, and tinctures.

Skullcap in blue: The scientific name for skullcap, Scutellaria lateriflora, often known as blue skullcap and American skullcap, has been linked to potential anti-anxiety properties. Early studies suggest that skullcap extract may have a soothing impact on an anxious person and create anxiety, despite the herb's modest efficacy findings. The leaves are consumed as tea and dust, as well as for medical purposes. Skullcap can occasionally cause liver function problems; therefore, it might not be appropriate for everyone.

Bonus Advice: Natural Sprays Investing in lavender and other natural linen sprays is another way to improve the quality of your sleep overall. For a scent that lasts longer, spray some on the bed as well as the linens and pillows.

You can use the herbal linen spray even outside of your pillow. Some of them can be sprayed on the curtains and drapes as well. You should order a carpet from Wovenly Rugs if your bedroom doesn't already have one. They can pick from a wide variety.

Choose a Nectar Mattress instead of popular herbal sleep aids like lavender for pleasant sleep to help you obtain the shut-eye you require.

A catuaba bark supplement is one of a group of herbal sleep aids that can gently and naturally assist in alleviating sleep issues. The benefit of employing a natural sleep herb is this: These days, melancholy and other sleep-related issues are rather common because many individuals struggle to fall asleep. Even though they are not common for anyone, sleep disruptions do happen. Males and females never have sleep issues at any age, as is natural. These are warning signs that something is amiss and needs to be fixed.

Where does catuaba bark come from?

A little tree called Errythroxylum catuaba is growing in northern Brazil. Like many painkiller herbs, it has the therapeutic power to soothe the nerves and lessen anxiety in general. Such preparations of this herbal sleep aid are perfect for making plans for a restful night.

This pill may still help if your discomfort prevents you from falling asleep because it is widely renowned for its pain-relieving properties. For a long time, people have relied on sleep aid medications to get the rest they need. Because there are so many factors that might disrupt sleep, sleep aids were widely used in ancient societies.

You only need to ask for an overview of the many situations and conditions that may interfere with regular sleeping patterns. Food allergies, stress, being overweight, feeling anxious all the time, and chronic exhaustion are just a few things that might make it difficult to get adequate sleep. The truth is that anything that may interfere with your ability to operate normally or with your general health could also affect how well you sleep.

Catuaba bark is a common sleep aid that aids in overcoming sleep difficulties so that you can have a good night's rest. It is an essential part of any medical therapy regimen intended to increase the quality and quantity of your sleep because of its ability to reduce general anxiety and emotional stress and control the numerous causes of insomnia.

You will be protected by catuaba bark extract from the dangers of lack of sleep. This member of the family of sleeping aid herbs will help you unwind in a manner that only a typical sleep herb can, whether it's to prevent the dangers of driving while fatigued or the health issues that result from extended periods of poor sleep.

Catuaba bark extract is one of the herbs that might help you sleep better at night by acting as a natural sedative. Lack of sleep first causes symptoms like fatigue and irritation, and if issues persist, they may cause impaired capacity to perform. Herbal sleep remedies will help you break the pattern and relax, so you can work and relax effectively.

Herbal sleep aids Some herbal remedies may be more effective than others at treating insomnia and sleep disorders. You should keep in mind that even herbs might be harmful if utilized improperly while treating any herbal illness. To be safe, always seek medical advice, especially if you are currently taking another medicine. The effects of various medications on each other could never be known. Try these sleeping herbs to ease your insomnia and restless nights after being cleared up by a doctor.

Triya Nanavati

PART 10

MEDICINAL HERBS TO FIGHT INFLAMMATION

The body uses inflammation as a critical mechanism to maintain healthy immunological function and to encourage the production of white blood cells. Why is it necessary to stop this, then? When the system is out of balance, this desire arises and, even in the absence of external threats, sets off an inflammatory response that damages the body's own tissues. You would undoubtedly need to live in a bubble, free of worry, sugar, saturated fats, and other environmental pollutants, to avoid this condition. Since this is not practical, you may ration it all out by including antioxidants and anti-inflammatory foods in your diet. We've included a number of spices and herbs below that work to reduce inflammation.

Turmeric: If there was ever a spice that could have been referred to as an all-arounder, it would have been turmeric. Its potent antioxidant, anti-inflammatory, antiviral, antibacterial, antifungal, and anticancer properties have made it a staple in Chinese and Indian medicine and cuisine for millennia. The curcumin molecule in the spice, along with a variety of other anti-inflammatory substances, is what gives it its beneficial properties.

Ginger: This spice has proven to be incredibly useful in the treatment of inflammation because it contains the gingerols shogaol and paradol, which inhibit the formation of free radicals like peroxynitrite. Ginger is also beneficial for pain treatment, providing relief from sore throats, muscular pains, and discomfort in general.

Cloves: This antioxidant-rich spice is excellent for controlling the body's generation of reactive oxygen species. Cloves also include kaempferol flavonoids and rhamnetin, which inhibit excessive oxidation, in addition to their primary component, eugenol, which inhibits the swelling of the COX-2 enzyme.

Rosemary: This herb not only makes food taste better, but it also monitors possible free radicals, such as superoxide, and stops the synthesis of prostaglandins, which are responsible for inflammation. To prevent the oil from oxidizing while cooking, rosemary may be added.

Cayenne pepper: Known for its spicy flavor and therapeutic properties, cayenne pepper has been employed by Indian, Chinese, and Native American healers for thousands of years. While the chemical components that make up capsaicin are responsible for the majority of its therapeutic effects, it also contains a number of flavonoids and carotenoids that work as antioxidants against free radicals to reduce inflammation.

Cinnamon: This spice is well-known for lowering blood sugar levels, but it also has a lot of other benefits. It has a variety of anti-inflammatory and antioxidant compounds that guard against inflammatory diseases and heart disease. inhibits the production of NF-kappaB proteins, which are responsible for inflammatory genes as well as blood platelet clustering.

Sage: Carnosic acid and carnosol, two anti-inflammatory compounds responsible for the sage's scent and therapeutic properties, are abundant in the plant's fragrant leaves. Due to exacerbated inflammatory responses, these substances provide defense against brain diseases like Alzheimer's. Additionally, this plant has anti-oxidant and anti-cancer components.

Thyme, a plant that is frequently used to season meat, is a treasure trove of healing compounds, including bioflavonoids and volatile oils like thymol. Thymol, the compound that gives thyme its antioxidant qualities, is also a potent antiseptic and antibacterial agent.

The truth is that herbs and spices, like the ones indicated above, contain lower quantities of these free radical scavengers than fruits and vegetables, despite the fact that most people are aware of this. So, add these spices to your meal and treat your ailment with flavor if you want to prevent inflammation or combat an existing problem.

PART 11

HERBAL TREATMENT TO RELIEVE STRESS

Herbs for anxiety are becoming considerably more common. The availability of herbal medicines has increased, from specialty teas to pills and capsules. There are several methods for overcoming stress, and dealing with anxiety may be a very challenging undertaking.

For a wide range of stress-related indications or symptoms, many people are seeking natural stress and anxiety remedies rather than standard medications. Medicines seem to be the best option for minimizing the negative effects of stress on the body since they help relax a hyperactive mind, reduce stress brought on by the accumulation of hazardous toxins, assist in breaking down anxiety, and enhance the heart and respiratory functions. Which are all constantly threatened by stress and worry.

These healing herbs have been used for about 5,000 years. They were utilized as medicines by the ancient Romans, Greeks, Egyptians, and especially the Chinese. Nowadays, using natural herbs as a stress reliever is a quick and frequently affordable solution.

A very helpful plant in the treatment of stress is Siberian ginseng. It can boost energy levels as well as cause irritation. By enhancing the neurological system, it can lessen mental and physical tiredness, treat melancholy and anxiety, and enhance pressure tolerance.

A well-known Indian herb called ashwagandha has been used for thousands of years to combat stress. It is an active herb that improves our capacity to deal well with internal and external causes of stress as well as change. It's especially helpful if you're worn out. This functions as an anti-inflammatory agent and boosts energy levels. In times of stress, Ashwagandha's anti-inflammatory effects are highly helpful since unneeded stress will increase systemic inflammation.

The key herb for pressure is Rhodiola rosea. Additionally, it aids in overcoming weariness, which improves focus and memory. It also activates the immune system, which aids in the defense against illness and infection.

Due to their occasionally negative side effects, many of us choose not to use prescription medications. The use of valerian root may be quite beneficial for treating insomnia. When administered before bed, it soothes the nerves and has a calming effect.

Finally, chamomile, a plant that is growing, can lower the pressure. Because of its calming effects, this is one of the most popular pressure herbs. It is one of the most widely used and easily accessible therapies to relieve depression when consumed as a cup of herbal tea. Additionally, it has sedative properties that promote restful sleep.

Using organic herbal medicines to relieve stress has a variety of ramifications. They are often mild, commonly available, affordable, and safe. Some pressure medications can be consumed in a variety of ways, including liquids, teas, tablets, and capsules. You may get any of them at the drugstore, a health food shop, or online. The safest person to seek advice from, as with all therapies, is a medical expert, especially if you have a pre-existing ailment or are on prescription medicine.

PART 12

MEDICINAL HERBS FOR HIGH BLOOD PRESSURE

The majority of individuals prefer the conventional approach to treating high blood pressure over high blood pressure medications. You have the advantage that many different herbs are quite effective in treating this widespread illness. Learn how to manage hypertension and improve your health using herbs for high blood pressure.

Today, a number of illnesses are successfully treated using herbs. No exception is made for treating high blood pressure. Herbs obviously don't have the same immediate impact as narcotics, but they can still be harmful over time. Additionally, herbs are safer and have no negative side effects.

Many individuals decide to treat their hypertension with herbs. If high blood pressure is not treated, it might result in heart attacks or strokes. Despite the existence of hypertension, anything greater than 120–139 systolic and 80–89 diastolic might be dangerous and has to be reduced.

Initially, there are typically no symptoms, but as the pressure rises, the patient may experience weariness, headaches, and nosebleeds. Although there is no one cause of hypertension, being overweight, eating too much salt, experiencing stress, and abusing alcohol can all significantly raise blood pressure.

To reduce the need for pharmaceuticals, there are several herbal medication combinations for high blood pressure as well as natural supplements that may be used: Garlic supplements are known to lower blood pressure, according to tests. Garlic should only be taken when taking blood thinners like aspirin or warfarin, however, and only under the guidance of a qualified medical professional.

Hawthorn—used by pharmaceutical companies, it has shown to be quite effective. When used in conjunction with blood pressure medicines, there have been no recorded adverse drug or herb effects.

Indian curry spice turmeric has anti-inflammatory, cholesterol-lowering, antioxidant, and blood vessel-improving properties in addition to lowering blood pressure.

Gingko biloba, a Chinese plant used to treat hypertension, improves blood flow and widens arteries. Additionally, memory and mental attentiveness are improved.

One of several herbs for high blood pressure, olive leaf supplements can treat arrhythmia, which is an erratic heartbeat.

From the Chinese mushroom family, maitake. As a result, ldl is reduced, and systolic and diastolic tensions are reduced.

Due to the inclusion of DHA and EPA fatty acids, which have been demonstrated to significantly enhance heart health, omega-3 essential fatty acids found in linseed oil and cod liver oil may be even better than fish oil.

Fish oil—Although it can only have a little impact, the DHA in fish oil helps to decrease blood pressure.

Dietary potassium, magnesium, and calcium are crucial for decreasing blood pressure.

Eating a nutritious diet that is rich in fresh fruit and vegetables is the best way to lower blood pressure. To reduce LDL cholesterol, cook with extra virgin olive oil and garlic. Consume less trans fat while increasing your intake of whole foods like nuts and grains.

Although using these natural treatments may be beneficial, it may also be necessary to combine them with prescription medications and a balanced diet, as advised. Additionally, the workout regimen should be followed. Exercise boosts metabolism and the flow of blood. It is crucial to speak with a doctor before quitting the use of prescription medications or taking any herbs for hypertension.

PART 13

HERBS FOR ARTHRITIS

Herbs for arthritis are many. It is true that arthritis may not be curable. However, they will significantly lessen the pain and inflammation that arthritis sufferers often experience. If everything else fails, you may find that these herbs are an excellent choice for you. The following are a few possible herbal remedies: Nettle Leaves: Nettle nettle is promoted as a natural alternative to NSAIDs. This herb's anti-inflammatory properties lessen arthritis-related swelling. The plant also includes boron, a vitamin that is suggested for those with arthritis. You can eat it or make tea with it.

In actuality, the name "Devil's Claw" comes from the appearance of its fruits, which resemble claws. It is a plant that grows throughout Africa and is well known for its capacity to reduce inflammation and discomfort. It is also thought to aid arthritis sufferers in improving joint mobility.

As much as you enjoy the flavor of ginger, its anti-inflammatory properties will make you appreciate it even more. Additionally, it can aid in easing discomfort. People who enjoy ginger a lot frequently claim that it seems to have no negative side effects. Ginger can be added to drinks or consumed as tea.

Celery is a common household ingredient that can be used to treat arthritis. This plant was also introduced to North America by contemporary European settlers. The plant contains potassium molecules and anti-inflammatory compounds that are advantageous to arthritis sufferers.

Red pepper is a necessary addition to the list of arthritis-relieving plants. This is undoubtedly one of the most popular natural pain relievers that is effective even for people without arthritis. The compound capsaicin, which gives peppers their characteristically fiery flavor, can also help reduce the sense of pain. Additionally, it causes the body to create more endorphins, which act as natural painkillers.

Its high nutritional content is this herb's main asset in the treatment of arthritis. Additionally, it helps to lessen fluid retention. Patients with arthritis are advised to drink this herb's tea. Alfalfa powder may aggravate arthritic symptoms.

Angelica-Dong quai is another name for this herb's species that is widely used. This plant is used to treat arthritis-related joint discomfort. This plant may be consumed as tea, just like other herbs.

Other herbs have anti-inflammatory and pain-relieving properties. The usefulness of herbs will be attested to honestly by those who handle them properly and appropriately. You should remember to keep safety in mind at all times. When used with specific medications, some herbs can have negative and sometimes harmful side effects.

Additionally, there are no set doses or combinations for herbs. Different sources and herbal specialists will have various opinions. It makes sure that there is no guarantee that a certain dose recommendation will work properly for you.

Herbs shouldn't be consumed without a doctor's prescription. The best way to take medications for arthritis is with your doctor's approval.

PART 14

HERBS FOR OTHER COMMON DISEASES

According to some experts, frequently consuming cranberry juice may prevent urinary tract infections (UTIs).

According to the National Institute of Diabetes and Digestive and Kidney Diseases, urinary tract infections, which are brought on by intestinal bacteria, are the second most frequent ailment in the body and are the reason for around 8.1 million medical visits each year. Women experience UTIs more frequently than men do. Doctors often advise utilizing modest dosages of the antibiotic administered for a period of six months or longer in patients with persistent UTIs.

Other compounds produced by cranberries are thought to prevent germs like Escherichia coli from colonizing the lining of the urinary system.

The researchers examined 24 trials with a total of 4,473 individuals for an analysis that was published in the Cochrane Database of Systematic Reviews' October 2012 issue. We found that cranberry juice was less effective than they had thought. When the findings of much bigger research were taken into account, the advantage for women with UTIs, although it had been demonstrated in several smaller trials included in the analysis, was not significant.

According to Dr. Anthony Schaeffer, Chairman of Northwestern Medicine Urology in Chicago, "certain evidence suggests that cranberry juice contains carbohydrates that can inhibit bacterial cell attachment, which is a crucial first phase in infection." But because it isn't strong enough, it doesn't seem to have an effect in the real world. Doctors advise patients to pee frequently and drink lots of water to prevent UTIs.

In a 2009 study that was published in Diabetic Medicine, researchers randomly assigned 58 people with type 2 diabetes to take cinnamon or a placebo for more than 12 weeks. They discovered that those who took two grams of cinnamon saw a 0.36 percent reduction in blood sugar levels. In contrast, those taking a placebo had a 0.13 percent rise in blood sugar levels. However, a recent assessment published in the September 2012 issue of the Cochrane Database of Systematic Reviews produced different findings. Cinnamon's impact on people with type 1 and type 2 diabetes was studied.

Between individuals who got cinnamon and those who received a placebo, there was no discernible difference in blood sugar levels. Menopause Warm menopausal flushes are frequently treated with red clover and black cohosh. Although there is no proof that standardized formulations are more effective than placebos, they are safe. In a tiny trial, compared to the control group, food and lifestyle advice and a customized herbal therapy improved libido and hot flashes in 15 individuals. Some diabetics use aloe vera to lower their blood sugar levels. Some diabetics utilize aloe vera to lower their blood sugar levels. Aloe vera, bilberry extract, bitter melon, ginger, cinnamon, and okra are among the natural plants and spices that many diabetics use to reduce blood sugar. Risks include the possibility that they may either not function, resulting in uncontrolled diabetes, or that they will work effectively but inconsistently, causing low blood sugar levels, particularly when used with other medications for decreasing blood sugar, such insulin.

Ayurvedic physicians integrate herbal remedies with lifestyle recommendations. Despite some encouraging findings and the absence of any major negative side effects, Cochrane's joint assessment of seven studies of Ayurvedic medications used to treat diabetes concluded that no conclusive conclusions could be reached. Up to a quarter of internet purchases of ayurvedic goods have been found to contain potentially hazardous quantities of metals, including lead, mercury, and arsenic. Asthma Some herbal treatments for asthma could be successful. An analysis of 17 randomized controlled trials for the use of Chinese and Ayurvedic medicine's herbal asthma therapies revealed a substantial improvement in more than half of the studies. Tylophora indica, cannabis, and dried leaf extract were among the herbs examined, although the research was unable to identify which of these was active. However, many botanicals have interactions with standard medical care. The symptoms of asthma may worsen because St. John's wort reduces the effectiveness of the asthma medication aminophylline. Among other things, royal jelly made by bees and sold by herbalists is used to treat asthma. However, Asthma UK strongly advises against using it since there have been cases of severe, and occasionally deadly, allergy and asthmatic reactions.

IBS, or irritable bowel syndrome To relieve the symptoms of diarrhea, bloating, and cramping associated with IBS, many patients with the condition resort to herbal remedies. There are formulations for rhubarb, mandarin, cardamom, and licorice, as well as five or more other plants, in traditional Chinese medicine. Although there is no research, UK doctors often give IBS patients peppermint oil capsules for bloating and cramps. Individual herbs can be utilized for specific symptoms. Ginger is typically thought to help with nausea, and there is some evidence that it works better than a placebo for morning sickness and motion sickness, albeit not necessarily in IBS. Iberogast, a blend of nine herbs and plant extracts, appears to be useful in relieving indigestion symptoms with few adverse effects.

Triya Nanavati

PART 15

MEDICINAL HERBS IN ORIENTAL TRADITION

As with other therapeutic modalities, the goal of oriental medicine is to treat the complete person. Eastern medicine therapies, including acupuncture, herbal medicine, acupressure, tuina, and other traditional Chinese medicine (TCM) applications, have been around since the birth of modern civilization to balance the mind, body, and spirit. In actuality, Easter medicine dates back about 5,000 years before the birth of Christ.

Modern Eastern medicine practitioners frequently combine natural healing modalities such as acupuncture, Tai Chi, moxibustion, cupping, and Chinese herbal therapy with dietary advice to treat patients.

Oriental medicine's use of acupuncture is predicated on the idea that the body has meridians, sometimes referred to as energy channels. These meridians include "acupoints" that control the movement of "chi," or life force. The idea behind this Asian medical procedure is that underlying pathologies (health disorders) can be alleviated by putting tiny, hair-like needles into these acupoints. Why is that so? The theory is that by inserting needles (at the appropriate acupoints), obstructions are removed, allowing the Chi to circulate freely and unhindered across the meridians. This is thought to balance life's power and restore the body's harmony and wellness.

Some Oriental doctors use a special type of acupuncture called auriculotherapy. Acupuncture needles are inserted along the meridians that run along the outer ear in this specific needling method. This therapy is frequently provided by acupuncturists who have received specialized training and certification.

Moxibustion or tapping therapy are additional treatments offered by practitioners of oriental medicine. In moxibustion, the plant "mugwort," or moxa, is utilized. The herbal medicine is combined with the acupoints, or the tips of the acupuncture needles, after being crushed and burned. The herbal medicine aims to warm these areas and encourage better chi flow.

In Oriental medicine, cupping is a treatment in which a cup (or cups) are used to create suction on the skin. When starting a fire, fire or flames are frequently briefly applied to the interior of the cup or cups before being applied to the body. On the body, it creates a suction resembling a vacuum. To encourage healing and pain alleviation, Chinese medicine practitioners might move the cup from one acupoint to another.

Simply enough, this method is called "gliding." Tai Chi and Qigong are two more natural healing exercises that doctors of oriental medicine may recommend to their patients. Tai Chi is a slow-moving martial art that has been shown to have stress-relieving properties. Additionally, it is a fantastic approach to developing joint and muscle flexibility and range of motion. Tai chi and qigong are frequently combined as breathing exercises to enhance and preserve health.

It is vital to investigate the credentials of the potential Oriental medicine doctor, just as with any other healthcare provider. Eastern medicine specialists like acupuncturists should have a license to practice in the state where they live. These practitioners must be certified by the National Certification Commission for Acupuncture and Oriental Medicine (NCCAOM) in order to apply for a license in several.

Eastern traditional medicine Chinese medicine, often known as traditional Chinese medicine (TCM), is a historical medical system that connects the laws and patterns of nature to the human body. TCM includes a wide range of techniques and has its roots in the more than 5,000-year-old Taoist philosophy.

One significant distinction between TCM and Western medicine is the relationship between the world and the human body. This point of view is based on the ancient Chinese conception of people as little representations of the larger, enclosing world who are connected to and susceptible to the forces of nature. The numerous organs, tissues, and other elements of the human body are regarded as an organic organism, each with a unique purpose but with strong interdependence. According to this viewpoint, the balance of functions affects both health and sickness.

TCM's focus on qi disruptions or vital energy in its diagnostic methods is another distinction between it and western medicine. In order to make a diagnosis, a doctor must observe (particularly their tongue), hear, smell, inquire, interview, and touch and palpate (especially their pulse).

Nei Jing (Inner Canon of the Yellow Emperor), a treatise of traditional Chinese medicine, details important ideas from TCM's theoretical underpinnings, including the idea of Yin-Yang, or the idea that the universe and all life are shaped by two opposing but complementary forces. Qi is the life force or vital energy that governs a person's physical, mental, emotional, and spiritual wellness. Along channels known as meridians, qi travels throughout the body and is changed by yin and yang. Maintaining harmony and balance in qi circulation is a lifelong effort that results in health. Eight guidelines, including yin/yang, indoor/outdoor, excess/deficiency, and cold/heat, are used to classify diseases and examine symptoms. Each of the five elements—fire, earth, metal, water, and wood—relates to a different organ or tissue in the body, and they all help to explain how the body functions.

Individualized care is a key component of traditional Chinese medicine. Acupuncture, herbal remedies, acupressure, qi gong, eastern massage, and tai chi are some of the treatment options. The fundamental tenet of traditional Chinese medicine is that the disease's origin, not its symptoms, should be treated.

The practice of traditional Chinese medicine dates back thousands of years in China. Often referred to as "traditional Chinese medicine," practitioners utilize herbs, diet, acupuncture, cutting, and qigong to prevent or cure health issues.

It is known that traditional Chinese medicine is a form of alternative medicine in the United States, despite the fact that modern medicine is still practiced in many medical facilities in China.

health advantages Western academics have not yet done a thorough study of how traditional Chinese medicine is used to treat particular illnesses. However, the following ailments are dealt with by traditional Chinese medicine: Allergies Anxiety Arthritis (like rheumatoid arthritis, for instance) Depression Pain, diabetes, psoriasis, eczema, acne, and other skin problems The diagnosis in contemporary medicine is based on conventional Chinese medicine. For instance, an insomniac may experience sleep problems as a result of imbalances such as renal or kidney failure, spleen insufficiency, or a blood shortage.

The unique approach

Taoism, a philosophy, is the foundation of traditional Chinese medicine, which was developed on the tenet that all bodily parts support one another. A person's organs (and their respective jobs) must be in balance for them to be healthy. One approach to achieving this harmony is to balance the opposing yet complementary forces of yin and yang, which are supposed to have an effect on all life. Another theory in traditional Chinese medicine is that the qi or chi, commonly known as the body's life force, moves via distinct pathways known as meridians. According to this theory, when the qi flow is impeded, weak, or excessive, diseases and other problems with one's emotional, mental, or physical health appear. The flow of qi must be resumed for yin and yang to be balanced and, consequently, for wellbeing to be attained.

What to expect

A practitioner of traditional Chinese medicine would evaluate your general health during a normal consultation by taking your medical history, analyzing your language, taking your pulse, and performing a physical examination. The examination would reveal any qi obstructions or imbalances.

The presence of an imbalance in one of the TCM organ systems does not always indicate that the patient has a medical ailment in that organ, according to the expert.

For instance, the liver aids in controlling the flow of qi. It is believed that when a person has "liver stagnation," their vitality is obstructed, resulting in symptoms like irritation, rage, or despair, a bitter aftertaste, indigestion, and a pulse that experts describe as "nervous."

But "yin renal failure" is also characterized by memory loss, tinnitus, hot flushes in the afternoon or evening, and dry mouth. The tongue often has little to no coating and is reddish in color. The pulse is described by practitioners as "floating."

Treatment methods

Acupuncture is the most widely utilized therapeutic technique in traditional Chinese medicine. The focus of traditional Chinese medicine is on tailored therapy; therefore, each patient receives care quite differently. These techniques frequently include:

Acupuncture is employed as a Western therapy for a number of health issues, despite its roots in traditional Chinese medicine.

Acupressure is the application of finger pressure to acupuncture sites and meridians.

Diet and nutrition: Food is said to have special therapeutic capabilities as well as heating and cooling effects.

TCM Herbs

Traditional Chinese medicine practitioners typically blend many different herbs in special formulas according to the needs of each patient rather than prescribing a singular herb. These mixtures can be taken as teas, pills, tinctures, or powders. The following plants are frequently employed in traditional Chinese medicine:

- astragalus
- Ginkgo biloba
- red rice yeast
- cinnamon
- ginger
- ginseng
- Gotu Kola
- Yu Xing Cao

Due to a lack of regulation, customers are exposed to dangers when purchasing food supplements (such as the possibility of contamination with other chemicals), but these hazards may be higher with foreign herbal goods, particularly those that contain a range of plants.

TCM may provide certain people with a special viewpoint on lifestyle choices that may have an impact on their health. There aren't many high-quality clinical investigations that demonstrate TCM's ability to treat diseases. Therefore, it's crucial to avoid using it in place of basic treatment or treating yourself.

If you're considering attempting traditional Chinese medicine, speak with an expert and your doctor to weigh the benefits and drawbacks of the treatment and decide if it's suitable for you.

Triya Nanavati

PART 16

FRESH HERBS AND DRIED HERB

The most precious components of every culture have been regarded as herbs and spices since the birth of civilization. Herbs enhance the flavor of food, making it taste considerably better than it otherwise would. Although chefs and cooks may now season meals using dried spices, it is still crucial to understand the distinction between fresh and dried herbs. Understanding the differences is crucial whenever there is one.

When compared to the prolonged time needed to use potted plants, spices and dried herbs quickly season meals. The majority of spices and herbs are conveniently available at specialty food stores.

Most recipes work well with these dried herbs and spices, and they are essential to a particular cuisine. Additionally, these dried herbs can be used to make herbal drinks. It is exceedingly challenging to locate fresh herbs and spices as compared to dried herbs. The majority of stores sell popular herbs like basil, oregano, rosemary, tarragon, parsley, chives, and dill in dry form, although they are quite pricey. These herbs are sometimes sold in potted form so that a proficient cook can always have access to them. Fresh herbs typically have a strong aroma and enhance the flavor of food.

Remember that dried herbs and spices may be used straight from the jar, whether you choose fresh or dried herbs. A bit more planning is necessary for great versions. Cooks should roast or crush spices like cumin and cardamom before using them in recipes. Some herbs, including basil, oregano, and rosemary, are available in fresh form and require adequate crushing and washing of the stems. Some herbs, like rosemary, don't require cutting. Hash must be prepared; however, the size should vary according to the meal. While the rosemary leaves can be left intact, the rosemary stem should be completely removed.

Additionally, the chef has the option of cultivating his own herb garden. While certain herbs are best utilized fresh, some can also be used dried. Herbs in pots may be purchased in stores and should be put close to windows with natural light for easy access. The choice between fresh and dried herbs is then theirs to make. Herbs can be dried in two ways: indoors in a dehydrator or outside in the sun.

The cook and gardener should regularly replenish their dried grass. Despite lasting longer than fresh herbs, they could eventually lose their taste. Herbs that have lost their taste in dry form should be thrown away and replaced later.

The price and restricted availability of fresh herbs and spices are their key distinctions. But the flavor it produces is unmatched. Since they are crucial for inventive cuisine, it is the responsibility of experienced chefs to select the best ones.

The majority of the time, herbs are plants' leaves. They have been utilized for many reasons over the years, particularly in cooking and healing. Herbs, both fresh and dried, give meals an unusual flavor when they are used in cooking. In many kitchens, discussions about dried and fresh herbs frequently result in questions. The way ingredients are stored, whether they are supplemented with herbs or not, and the cooking procedure all affect how a dish tastes. You'll find some advice in this post to guide your choice between using dried and fresh herbs.

Use this standard conversion if you wish to swap fresh herbs for dried herbs. A tablespoon of fresh herbs is equivalent to a teaspoon of dry grass when added. Be cautious not to overcook if you plan to cook something for several hours so that the herbs' tastes can come through. Additionally, the chef has the option to add fresh or dried herbs once the meal has finished cooking. You should do the reverse if you are cooling food, such as pasta salads, for instance. When seasonings are applied in advance, the meal has a really unique flavor.

While comparing dried and fresh herbs, look for variations in price and accessibility. The cook should treat fresh herbs like fresh flowers when purchasing them. To begin, trim the stem at the base and get rid of any decaying leaves. The rest of the plant can be utilized with soft stems. The stems must be placed in a glass of water and protected with plastic wrap. Place the pan in the fridge and replace the water every day.

If you want to cultivate your own herbs, you can store them in the freezer after washing and drying them for a few months. Just put freezer bags with your fresh herbs inside. Plants like goblets, dill, basil, parsley, and chives freeze beautifully.

A common error is to keep dry herbs close to the oven. This is not advised since ongoing heat exposure would gradually destroy their flavor and scent. A similar outcome will be seen if you are exposed to too much sunshine. As a result, it is recommended to keep dried herbs in a cold, dark location.

The herbs can be dried in the microwave, which will save time. To begin, wash the herbs and spread them out on absorbent paper to dry. The herbs should then be heated for a little while in the microwave. Laurel leaves and marjoram are two herbs that can't stand being exposed to microwaves for an extended period of time.

After drying, you can finish the process by milling the herbs or drying them with your fingers. Dried herbs can also be tested for freshness by being rubbed between your fingers. Throw it out if it isn't aromatic.

Although fresh and dried herbs have certain characteristics, both kinds have a place in each kitchen's cupboard and freezer.

Great Ways To Dry Fresh Herbs

You spent a lot of time tending to your herb garden, and it paid off by giving you more herbs than you could possibly utilize. What do you do with extra herbs now that you don't utilize them all?

The drying of your herbs becomes apparent at this point. Currently, drying fresh herbs is not difficult, but in order to ensure that the herbs you dry are the tastiest possible, you must be aware of the available drying processes and suitable harvesting procedures.

Harvesting Medicinal Plants

Depending on the species of grass and the place where it is cultivated, there are several ideal times to harvest the herb.

Herbs often use more energy to develop flowers and seeds than leaves, so it is ideal to pick them before they blossom to preserve their leaves.

If you pick up your dried herbs after you start sprouting blooms, they will have lost much of their taste.

Now, choosing leaves—which are most frequently used in cooking—confirms that this basic rule is typically valid. If the leaves are not what you are searching for, however, this rule no longer applies.

The best time to harvest the stems is when the plant begins to bloom, and the best time to pick the blooms is just before blooming.

Prior to using the herbs, make sure to properly clean and rinse the leaves and stems of the herbs.

Plant drying techniques

Herbs can be dried using a variety of methods. Depending on how many plants you dry, the space you have, and how long you wait for the plants to dry, you'll need to decide which strategy to employ.

Stop drying

The method, which is often referred to as air drying or bag drying, is excellent for grasses with many stems. The goal is to group the herbs into manageable bunches and secure the stems with ribbons. It is a good idea to mark the herbs before drying to help identify them, so there is no confusion on the road after drying. The majority of dried herbs look like this.

Each herb bag should be placed in a small paper bag with the top of the package facing the bag. Pack the item in a dry, well-ventilated area after kneading the bag's opening around the stem.

Because it permits all the nutrients and flavor found in the plant stems to penetrate the leaves, this process yields the tastiest dried herbs. On the other hand, it takes the longest to dry herbs, taking somewhere between one and three weeks.

Screen drying

Small plants benefit greatly from this method. Your herbs can be placed on the window sill or the gauze that has been put out on the frame. Keep your herbs out of the sun and in a dry area. To ensure that they dry evenly, be sure to mix them every other day. The herbs may normally be dried using this method in approximately a week.

Oven drying

Using this method, you want to separate the leaves from the stem and arrange them on a baking sheet in a uniform layer. As soon as the herbs are tender, flip them every 20 to 30 minutes in the lowest position in the oven. The temperature is too high if you can smell herbs while the food is baking. If the oven cannot be turned off, you can leave the door slightly ajar. Depending on the thickness of the leaves, this process might take anywhere between three and five hours.

Microwave drying

The fact that I prefer more organic methods of drying herbs is the only reason I'm not a great fan of this method. However, this method can work for you if you don't have much time to wait for your herbs to dry. The leaves should once again be separated from the stem and placed on a paper towel.

Cook for roughly 30 seconds in the microwave. This makes it easy to burn your herbs, so take care not to overcook them. Of course, use your pan, but after two to three minutes, your herbs should be dry.

Storage of dried herbs

You must get your herbs ready for storage after they have dried. Herb powders work well in electric coffee grinders. Of course, you don't want to grind herbs and coffee in the same coffee grinder. Both won't taste as good as you expected. You may use a mortar and pestle or a hand grinder to crush herbs.

Put your herbs in labeled containers and keep them out of the sun in a closet so they can last up to a year.

Triya Nanavati

Microwave drying

The fastest method of curing is the microwave drying, but this works only if you are in a great rush or if this method fits into your lifestyle. This method is obvious for you if you don't have fresh time to wait for your herbs to dry. The leaves or sprigs to be suggested from the stem and placed in a paper towel.

Cook for 1 minute, periodically flipping and turning. This makes it easy to bring your herbs, so take care not to overcook them. Of course, the overall goal, but after two to three minutes, your herbs should be dry.

Storage of dried herbs

You must keep your herbs in dry storage after drying. A direct Herb crowding works well. Electric coffee grinders, of course, will not want to grind broth, and coffee in the same bottle grinder, both won't fit as might be expected. You may use a mortar and pestle, and hand grinder to crush herbs. But you have a handed container and keep them out of the sun in a cool so they can last up to a year.

82

PART 17

ESSENTIAL OILS

Essential oils are highly concentrated plant extracts that are used for their therapeutic properties. A range of plant parts, such as leaves, flowers, stems, roots, and fruits, are generated by cold pressing or distillation. Essential oils have been utilized for thousands of years and are still frequently used today because of their medicinal properties.

There are many different types of essential oils, each with unique features and benefits. Lemon, lavender, peppermint, tea tree, and eucalyptus essential oils are the ones that are used the most frequently. While lavender is well known for its calming and relaxing qualities, peppermint is frequently utilized for its energizing and stimulating properties. While tea tree oil is commonly used for its antibacterial and antifungal properties, eucalyptus is frequently utilized for its respiratory benefits. Lemon oil is known for having revitalizing and energizing properties.

Aromatherapy, topical use, and ingestion are some of the many uses for essential oils. Aromatherapy uses essential oils to improve both physical and emotional well-being through inhalation. A few drops of the oil can be added to a diffuser or inhaled directly from the bottle to achieve this. When using essential oils topically, they are applied directly to the skin, typically after being mixed with a carrier oil like coconut oil or almond oil. It is possible to utilize essential oils by eating them internally, but it's important to keep in mind that not all essential oils are suitable for consumption and that you should only do this with your doctor's permission.

Essential oils may enhance digestion and fortify the immune system, in addition to promoting relaxation and reducing stress. For example, lavender oil may be used to promote relaxation and improve the quality of sleep. Peppermint oil can be used to alleviate headaches and promote mental clarity. Tea tree oil can be used as a natural remedy for acne and other skin problems. Eucalyptus oil can be used to treat respiratory issues, including coughing and congestion. You may use lemon oil to lift your spirits and emit a delicate perfume.

When using essential oils, it's critical to do it safely and intelligently. Essential oils should always be diluted before use due to their high potency. It's also suggested to perform a patch test before applying an essential oil to the skin because some people may react unfavorably. Essential oils must also be carefully stored and kept out of the reach of children and animals.

In addition to their medical use, essential oils may be used in a variety of household and cosmetic products. Lavender oil may be used to give laundry detergent a natural scent, while peppermint oil can be used to flavor homemade toothpaste. While eucalyptus oil may be used to infuse a steam shower with a spa-like ambience, tea tree oil can be used to cure dandruff in shampoo. Lemon oil may be added to cleaning products to give them a fresh scent and to help clean surfaces.

Although using essential oils to improve health and wellness may be a safe and useful method, they shouldn't be used in place of expert medical advice or care. Without the guidance of a knowledgeable healthcare professional, essential oils should not be used to treat or cure any medical condition. They must only be used in conjunction with standard medical care.

Other things to think about while using essential oils include the following:

Quality is crucial. Selecting pure, quality oils free of contaminants or additives is vital since not all essential oils are created equally. Select reputable businesses that acquire their oils from reputable suppliers and employ independent testing to ensure the purity and quality of their products.

Since essential oils are highly concentrated, they should always be diluted before use. Dilution of essential oils with a carrier oil promotes dispersion of the oil over a wider area in addition to reducing the potential for skin sensitivity or irritation. Standard essential oil and carrier oil dilution ratios range from 1% to 2%; however, they might vary depending on the oil and the application.

It is possible to utilize essential oils for emotional support. Essential oils may significantly improve our mental health in addition to their many physical benefits. Aromatherapy with essential oils may help with stress relief, mood enhancement, and relaxation. Some oils, like bergamot and frankincense, are particularly helpful for emotional support.

Some essential oils should not be applied to animals. Others can be dangerous to animals, even if some essential oils may be a natural way to assist human health and wellness. Peppermint, tea tree, and eucalyptus are a few essential oils that are particularly prone to irritation. Unless specifically told to do so by a professional, ask your veterinarian before using essential oils directly on or around your pets.

Since essential oils and medicines may interact, it's critical to be informed of any potential interactions before using either. Some oils, including bergamot and grapefruit, may interfere with a drug's metabolism and cause undesirable side effects. Always check with your doctor before using any essential oils if you are on any medications.

Essential oils may be used for natural cleaning and disinfecting duties around the house in addition to their medical use. Tea tree, lemon, and eucalyptus oils are all effective for sanitizing and cleaning surfaces. They may be used in homemade cleaning products or in diffusers to purify the air.

Some essential oils may be used as a natural flavoring in baking and cooking and are safe to ingest. Additionally, essential oils can be used in cosmetics. You should only use oils that are marked as "safe for consumption" to be on the safe side. Popular cooking oils include orange, lemon, and peppermint.

Using essential oils for skin and hair care may be advantageous. The skin and hair benefit from the benefits of several essential oils. Tea tree oil is effective against dandruff and acne, while lavender oil soothes irritated or inflamed skin. It is well known that rosemary oil encourages the growth of healthy hair and scalp. It is vital to dilute essential oils and do a patch test to check for allergic reactions before applying them to the skin or hair.

By adding essential oils to the massage oil or lotion, the therapeutic effects of massage may be amplified. While lavender and chamomile oils are calming and soothing, eucalyptus and peppermint oils may provide relief for sore muscles and joints.

Citronella, lavender, and peppermint are a few essential oils that may help ward off insects and other pests. Natural pest control may be accomplished by using essential oils. They may be used to make homemade bug spray or put in a diffuser to keep off insects.

In general, essential oils are a versatile and all-natural remedy that may be applied in a number of different ways to enhance health and wellbeing. It's critical to always act responsibly, attentively, and under the guidance of a healthcare professional while using essential oils for medical purposes. When used carefully and under supervision, essential oils may be a helpful addition to your health and wellness routine.

Triya Nanavati

CONCLUSION

Herbal medicine is regarded as a supplemental therapy that treats disease or damage using herbs and plant extracts. From sadness to the flu, there are several herbal treatments and medications to cure any ailment.

The majority of medicines, even expensive prescription medicines, are really derived from plants. For instance, the painkiller morphine is derived from poppy seeds, whereas aspirin is made from willow bark. Digitalis is the source of the heart rhythm medication digoxin.

Traditional herbal therapy is not the only way that plants may be used as medication. Another instance of how plants are used in complementary therapy is in Chinese herbal medicine. Instead of only treating the symptoms, herbal therapy treats the whole person, utilizing a holistic approach. He is attempting to aid the body's healing process.

Different plant components, such as the flowers, seeds, and leaves, can affect a person in various ways. Herbalists believe that in order to get the finest results, the delicate chemical balance of the entire plant is necessary. Herbal treatment makes no such attempts, in contrast to conventional medicine, which frequently seeks to extract or duplicate certain plant ingredients.

Although certain herbs can be helpful for specific health issues, this does not imply that all herbs are always safe for use. For instance, it's not advisable to use numerous herbs when pregnant.

Herbal drugs might have side effects or adverse drug interactions, just like any other medication. If you have issues with high blood pressure, glaucoma, or heart disease, you should start taking herbs under the supervision of a doctor. Additionally, herbal remedies should not be used to treat some life-threatening conditions, including epilepsy, type 1 diabetes, and others. When using herbs, never go beyond the stated dosage.

At health food shops, pharmacies, and even some supermarkets, you may buy alternative medicine herbs and medications in the form of tablets, capsules, ointments, creams, and pills. Despite the fact that they may be purchased over the counter, it is always a good idea to speak with a physician or herbalist, particularly if your condition is severe. If you are expecting or nursing, use herbs with great caution. Without first contacting your doctor, never switch your prescription medications. Numerous GPs will collaborate with plants.

Initial consultations with herbalists often last for at least an hour. Herbs, alternative medicinal practices, general health, and medical and family histories will all be covered during this consultation. Expect to be questioned about your previous and present emotional conditions as well as your lifestyle.

Changes in food and lifestyle, as well as the use of herbal supplements, are all possible when using herbs as an alternative form of treatment. It's possible that you'll be asked to bring a variety of plants that have been selected just for you. These supplements can come in tablet or capsule form, as well as syrup, lotion, tincture, gargle, inhaler, or washing solution form. You may make a follow-up appointment for a few weeks from now, and you can continue seeing an herbalist every month, depending on your condition and overall health.

I appreciate you taking the time to read this book. I have no doubt that you learned a lot from it because you now know which herbs work best for treating certain illnesses.

BONUS 1

TIPS FOR GROWING HERBS

Because there are so many different herbs to choose from, novice gardeners may find it difficult to decide which plants to grow. You may get a general concept of the varieties of herbs used in cooking and a planting guide for the herb garden by taking a short look at the shelf at your local grocery store.

The following list of herbs and tastes that are suitable for beginners includes:

Strong herbs - savory, rosemary, sage

Sweet basil, dill, mint, sweet marjoram, tarragon, and thyme are among the herbs that are potent enough to emphasize.

combining chives, parsley, and savory

You may increase the variety of herbs in your herb garden as your requirements and interests grow. When choosing herbs for the first time, keep in mind that they might be annuals, biennials, or perennials.

Annual (floral season, then death) basil, chervil, coriander, dill, anise, and savory

Biennials (two-season plants that only bloom in the second season) parsley, caraway

Once established, perennials (seasonally blooming) include savory, marjoram, tarragon, mint, chives, fennel, and love.

Tips for growing outdoor herbs

The northeast is where the most commonly used herbs grow. You may incorporate the herbs into your garden if you have the space. You can do everything better and be more organized with the square foot gardening approach, which we highly suggest. However, you might choose to cultivate herbs, particularly perennials, in a separate area.

Size of the herb garden

Determine the size of your herb garden first; it will depend on how much diversity you desire. A vegetable garden may typically be 20 feet by 4 feet in size. For distinct grasses, 12 x 18-inch individual plots in the region ought to be adequate. Some of the most vibrant and popular plants, including parsley and purple basil, may be grown as border plants. Keep perennials and annuals apart. It will also be helpful to have a map of the region and labels for the flora.

Site and soil condition

Drainage and soil richness should be taken into account when deciding where to put your herb garden. Probably the most crucial element for a successful crop is drainage. In damp soils, none of the grasses will grow. If the garden area is poorly drained, you will need to change the soil. Remove dirt from the garden plot to a depth of 15 to 18 inches to enhance drainage. At the bottom of the site that was dug, spread a 3-inch layer of crushed stone or a comparable substance. Mix compost or peat moss with the soil to soften the texture before returning it to the bed. The beds should then be filled to a level above the original to allow for soil sedimentation.

There is no need for the soil to be exceptionally productive at the location, so little fertilizer should be applied. Very rich soils typically yield an abundance of poor-quality leaves. The fertilizer needs for plants including chervil, fennel, coot, and savory are minimal. Per 100 square feet of garden space, adding several bushels of peat or compost can help the soil become healthier and hold onto moisture.

Sow seeds of herbs

The seeds of almost all herbs can be planted. Rust affects money, while relatively few illnesses or insects affect grass. Red mites can be seen on low-growing plants during hot, dry weather. Aphids may affect fennel, dill, caraway, and anise.

Some plants, like mint, must be kept under check lest they overgrow a garden. They should be planted in no. 10 cans or buckets with multiple drainage holes drilled slightly above the bottom edge. You might also use a clay pot, a drain, or a cement block. Put them in the ground; this should keep the plants contained for a while.

Additionally, herbs may be cultivated in planters, hanging baskets, pots, and square-foot gardening plots. These techniques will take more attention, particularly watering and a good location in the sun.

At the end of winter, if at all feasible, spread the seeds in small boxes. In the spring, transplant seedlings outside. The seedlings grow best indoors in bright, well-drained soil. Take care not to screw it up.

Most 2-year-olds must manually put seeds into the ground in the late spring. The soil surface should be given a fine texture and a little misting of water. Close the earth around the seeds after planting them in extremely shallow rows. Avoid planting seeds too deeply. If you combine fine seeds with sand, such as marjoram, kimchi, or thyme, they will disperse more evenly. One-eighth inch of soil may be applied to some of the bigger seeds. When planting fine seeds, keep the soil damp during germination by covering the bed with wet jars or paper. Water was sprayed finely to stop dirt from rinsing.

Cup and Division-

Additionally, cutting and division are helpful in the multiplication of some plants. When seeds take a long time to sprout, cuttings can be the answer. Some plants, meanwhile, proliferated swiftly enough that division became their main method of dissemination. Divide the tarragon, chives, and mint while cutting the lavender.

Garden Lawn Plan: Simple Steps for Novices

There's no denying that. We now have larger veggies and better-shaped meats thanks to modern breeding and agricultural techniques, but how about the flavor?

So what should you do if you want to try to give your dish a bit more flavor? Follow the example set by our ancestors by regularly using herbs in your cuisine. Even the sweetest foods can be made exciting with the correct herbs, especially when they are fresh from your own herb garden.

Plan of the cook's herb garden

Making a plan is the first step in constructing your own kitchen plant garden, which is the topic of this essay. Once it has established itself, your herb garden will give you a plentiful supply of all the plants you desire that are easy to reach. If you've never grown herbs before, don't worry. Really, it's not that tough as long as you create the strategy outlined below.

I don't want to teach you all there is to know about farming herbs, but if you take the advice I gave, you will have a sound strategy and design that will serve as the foundation for growing herbs. You'll need every type of plant.

Four steps to create a garden plan

1. Choose your herbs

The first step is to decide which herbs you wish to plant. If you don't waste time considering it, you'll wind up growing some things you don't need and omitting certain culinary necessities.

There are 100 different plants that you may choose to incorporate into your strategy. While some thrive in sunny locations with well-drained soil, others like wetness and shade. A good general tip is to pick a sunny area. To arrange the plants you have chosen correctly in the garden you will create after drafting your design, you must, however, be aware of the optimal circumstances for each of the plants you have chosen.

Make a note of all the herbs you are familiar with or frequently use in cooking before picking any. List names first, but allow space for kind (annual or perennial), ideal location (sunny, shaded), and best soil conditions (well-drained, wet, etc.) to follow. Leave room to describe the height that each plant will reach.

Add more herbs to your list at this point. Sage, etragon, marjoram, basil, lemon thyme, chives, parsley, rosemary, bay leaf, garlic, mint, and thyme are the herbs that are most frequently used in cooking. To finish your list, you will need to conduct some research, but this is a crucial stage in creating your strategy. When your list is finished, it should contain the names of several plants as well as the other details I mentioned above.

2. Select a location and choose a plant garden design

In order to pick fresh herbs whenever you need them, your herb garden should ideally be close to the kitchen. Four by six feet is an excellent size for a garden. You should be able to use this to plant all of the herbs on your list, including some perennial grasses. Try to pick a spot that faces south. If some of the plants you select require shade, consider using bigger plants to provide it, such as berries, tarragon, and rosemary.

Rectangles are the most basic plant garden layout, but consider different layouts like "islands" and raised beds. Alternately, think about creating a long-grass garden (excellent if your garden has a sunny wall). Design selection may be a lot of fun. Try once again looking at other models online or at your local library.

3. Check the soil conditions

After deciding on a spot for your herb garden, you must assess the soil's quality. Rich, well-dug, well-drained soil is desirable, while certain plants prefer various circumstances. To improve your soil, you might need to remove a lot of organic debris. However, be sure that none of it contains weeds, particularly perennials. If this is the case, you may use your herbs to shoot weeds when you try to remove them after they begin to grow.

4. Draw your patio garden design

Create a schematic of your garden on paper (on square paper, if you have one, after selecting the layout of your plants). On a scale, draw. Make the garden's foot on paper equal to two inches.

Now, cut rough circles from paper in various colors to depict your mature plants. Use the same one- to two-inch scale for these circles, and they should have the same diameter as each plant's growing height. Make room for additional varieties of herbs you might like to grow, such as sage and basil. One bigger herb, such as bay leaf or rosemary, will do.

Place the cut circles in ideal locations for each plant on your paper ladder. Some people also take into account the color of the flowers the plants will bear, but I advise avoiding this complexity. You may simply shift your herbs to the next year after the vegetation is past (but stop moving perennials after that).

You will know just where to plant your herbs when you plan your herb garden. A helpful hint is to make life-size circles in colored sand and place them precisely where your herb garden would be. By doing this, you can be sure that you've placed your plants precisely where they need to be and that there is enough room around them for them to flourish. Remember to make an effort to consider the requirements of plants that require a bit more shade.

Your strategy will enable you to develop a lovely herb garden that has every plant you want for your kitchen. You'll probably want to alter a few of the annual plants you initially chose after your first year of herb planting. That's okay; cultivating plants is enjoyable in spite of this. Perhaps you want to add sculptures or decorations to your herb garden to make it more eye-catching and aesthetically pleasing.

Triya Nanavati

BONUS 2

THE 9 APHRODISIAC HERBS: UNVEILING THE SECRETS TO INTENSE PASSION!

Natural herbs have long been thought of as potential treatments for enhancing sexual life. These plants contain aphrodisiac qualities that can heighten libido, boost sexual desire, and enhance sexual performance. Let's look more closely at a few of the herbal remedies that are believed to have aphrodisiac properties and can enhance your sexual life.

Ginseng

Traditional Chinese medicine has traditionally used the herb ginseng to promote sexual wellness. A real sexual tonic, ginseng root is especially well known for its stimulating effects on the neurological system.

Ginseng's capacity to boost energy and enhance physical endurance is one of its key qualities. Those who want to enhance their sexual performance but feel weary or exhausted may find this extremely helpful. Regular ginseng use can help fight exhaustion and boost energy levels, giving you more vigor during sexual activity.

Additionally, ginseng may help men with erectile dysfunction by enhancing their sexual performance. This is in part because it can encourage the body to release nitric oxide. Nitric oxide is a substance that aids in relaxing blood vessels and enhancing blood flow. Stronger, longer-lasting erections can be achieved and maintained with the help of improved blood flow to the penis.

Studies have revealed that ginseng can also raise testosterone levels, which are essential for male sexual health. The hormone testosterone is essential for controlling fertility, erections, and sexual desire. Healthy sexual function can be facilitated by an optimal testosterone balance in the body.

Ginseng root extract pills can be used to help with sexual wellness. It's crucial to get a high-quality item from a dependable vendor and to adhere to the instructions provided on the packaging. When used in the authorized amounts, ginseng is usually regarded as safe, although it is always best to speak with a doctor before beginning any kind of supplement.

Maca

An Andean root called maca has been used for generations as a natural aphrodisiac and treatment for sexual dysfunction. This plant is indigenous to the highlands of Bolivia and Peru, where it has long been valued for its positive effects on both men's and women's sexual health.

The capacity of maca to increase libido and sexual function is one of its key characteristics. Numerous studies have demonstrated that taking maca regularly can boost sexual desire and enhance sexual performance. For people who might have low libido or diminished sexual desire, this is very crucial. In order to improve the synthesis of sex hormones like testosterone, which is essential for both men's and women's sexual health, maca works by activating the endocrine system.

Maca has aphrodisiac properties in addition to being nutrient-rich, which can aid with sexual wellness. It includes a variety of vitamins, minerals, and crucial amino acids that promote the body's healthy operation. Vitamin C, vitamin E, and B vitamins are all present in maca and are crucial for boosting immunity and enhancing general health. Maca also contains considerable levels of minerals, including calcium, iron, copper, and zinc, which might enhance sexual health. Maca may have beneficial effects on energy and mood in addition to its direct effects on libido and sexual performance. After using maca, many people report having more energy and feeling generally better. If you want to increase your sexual experience while feeling weary or exhausted, this might be extremely useful. Additionally, maca is well-known for its adaptogenic qualities, which can lessen tension and exhaustion and foster an atmosphere that is conducive to sexuality and pleasure.

You can consume maca as an extract, powder, or nutritional supplement. To guarantee optimal efficacy, it's critical to select high-quality items from reliable suppliers. Before using maca, like with any supplement or natural treatment, it is always essential to speak with a doctor, especially if you are on medication or have a history of medical issues.

Tribulus Terrestris

Traditional Chinese and Ayurvedic medicine have long used the herb Tribulus terrestris to increase libido and sexual potency. This plant, which is indigenous to many parts of the world, is well-known for its positive effects on both men's and women's sexual health.

The presence of steroidal saponins is one of the reasons Tribulus terrestris is regarded as a natural aphrodisiac. Numerous potential advantages of Tribulus terrestris for sexual health can be attributed to these chemical constituents. The body's testosterone levels can be raised by steroidal saponins. Testosterone is a crucial hormone for libido and sexual function in both men and women.

Sexual desire, sperm production, erection quality, and sexual potency are all significantly influenced by testosterone. For men to maintain healthy sexual health and optimal performance in bed, appropriate testosterone levels are crucial. In women, testosterone plays a role in promoting sexual desire and general sexual health.

Tribulus terrestris can encourage higher amounts of testosterone in the body when taken regularly. Numerous advantages for sexual health may result from this. For instance, one of the most frequent side effects of Tribulus terrestris use is an increase in libido. Many claim that after ingesting this herb, they have more desire and interest in becoming sexual.

Tribulus terrestris can help boost sexual potency in addition to libido. Having more testosterone can help you perform better in bed and have more sexual vigor and endurance. For both parties, this may result in more gratifying and pleasurable sexual interactions.

The benefits of Tribulus terrestris might, however, differ from person to person, so it's crucial to keep that in mind. Some people could gain more than others. Additionally, before commencing any supplements or herbal usage for sexual health, especially if you are on medication or have a pre-existing medical issue, it is imperative to speak with a doctor.

Ginkgo Biloba

A centuries-old plant, ginkgo biloba has a long history of usage in traditional Chinese medicine. Many people are aware of this plant's possible health advantages, which include enhancements to sexual performance. Improved blood circulation is one of the key ways Ginkgo biloba can impact sexual wellness.

Healthy blood flow is essential for sexual function, especially for males seeking to get and keep an erection. The genitals' blood flow may be significantly improved by ginkgo biloba. The active ingredients in this plant have the ability to widen blood vessels and enhance regional blood circulation. This implies that during sexual excitement, more blood may reach the penile tissues, resulting in a harder erection and more sexual sensitivity.

Ginkgo biloba is well-known for its antioxidant effects in addition to its ability to increase blood circulation. Antioxidants aid in preventing blood vessel aging and free radical damage. Long-term improved blood circulation may result from this since it helps keep blood vessels flexible and healthy. Sexual function and general health can benefit from better blood vessel health.

Ginkgo biloba may also have additional advantages for sexual health. For instance, according to some studies, this plant may aid in reducing inflammation and enhancing endothelial function, both of which are crucial for blood flow and vascular health. The neural system may benefit from Ginkgo biloba's favorable effects on stress and anxiety, which can impair sexual performance.

Before utilizing Ginkgo Biloba, like with any dietary supplement or herbal treatment, it's crucial to speak with a doctor. It's crucial to take into account any potential drug interactions or pre-existing medical issues. A doctor or other health care provider can offer specialized direction and counsel on the ideal dosage.

Damiana

The interesting and potent Mexican plant known as daivana has long been used as a natural aphrodisiac. This plant, which has the scientific name Turnera diffusa, was utilized by prehistoric Mesoamerican societies to enhance libido and sexual function.

Flavonoids, terpenes, and alkaloids like damianin are only a few of the active compounds found in damiana. Together, these ingredients stimulate the neurological system, giving you more vigor and energy. Nervous system stimulation can help boost libido and sexual desire, resulting in a more satisfying encounter in bed.

But Damiana's appeal as a sexual health herb extends beyond pleasure. On the body, it also offers amazing calming and relaxing benefits. These soothing effects can aid in lowering stress, anxiety, and tension, which frequently interfere with closeness and sexual enjoyment. Damiana can assist in creating the optimal setting for a satisfying personal experience. Relaxing and feeling comfortable are essential components of a healthy and joyful sexuality.

Damiana is renowned for its beneficial effects on the emotional and mental spheres as well. As a nerve tonic, it can lift one's spirits, lessen weariness, and enhance sensations of all-around wellbeing. A healthy, balanced emotional state can enhance sexual engagement and pleasure, resulting in a more gratifying interaction between the partners.

A popular natural cure for stress and anxiety relief is dahlia. Chronic stress and worry can harm sexual health by lowering arousal potential and limiting desire. Damiana's soothing and unwinding qualities can help lower tension and anxiety levels, fostering a setting that is conducive to pleasurable sexuality.

Although Damiana is generally regarded as safe for use, it is always suggested to speak with a healthcare provider before using it as a supplement. People who use drugs or have pre-existing medical disorders should pay particular attention to this. An expert can offer individualized guidance and information on the ideal dosage.

Muira Puama

An important Amazonian plant called Muira Puama has a long history of usage in traditional medicine as a stimulant and aphrodisiac. This plant, which has the scientific name Ptychopetalum olacoides, is well-known for its potential advantages for libido, sexual potency, and physical vitality.

For decades, muira puama has been used as an herbal treatment to enhance sexual performance. Its primary role is to increase pelvic blood flow, which is essential for a good erection. To achieve and sustain an erection, there must be enough blood flow to the penis. Muira Puama can support enhanced erectile function and greater sexual sensitivity by boosting blood flow to the genital tissues.

Additionally, Muira Puama could enhance the flow of oxygen to vaginal tissues. For sexual tissues to function properly and stay healthy, enough oxygen flow is essential. The plant may encourage greater sexual performance by encouraging enhanced oxygen flow to the genitals.

Muira Puama may improve physical vitality and overall health in addition to its effects on sexual function. It is well recognized for its energizing qualities, which can boost vigor and endurance. For people who want to increase their physical vigor or who are feeling worn out, this can be extremely helpful.

Several active substances, such as alkaloids, sterols, and essential oils, may be found in Muira Puama. The intended effects on sexual health and physical vitality are achieved by the synergistic action of these substances. A health care provider should always be included in the usage of Muira Puama as a supplement since the effects might differ from person to person.

Before using Muira Puama, like with any dietary supplement or herbal treatment, it is always essential to talk to a doctor. It is crucial to take into account any potential drug interactions or pre-existing medical issues. For the finest outcomes, a health expert can provide you with individualized advice on the right dosage and security of utilizing Muira Puama.

Ashwagandha

An Ayurvedic herb called Ashwagandha is well-known for its various advantages for health and energy, including sexual wellness. Because of this plant's adaptogenic characteristics, which aid in lowering stress and exhaustion in the body, ancient Indian medicine has treasured it for generations.

The capacity of ashwagandha to lessen stress is one of the primary reasons it is linked to enhanced sexual health. Chronic stress can have a deleterious impact on libido and sexual function, resulting in less arousal and desire. As an adaptogen, ashwagandha can assist the body in better managing stress and reestablishing hormonal equilibrium. This may help with greater sexual response and increased sexual desire.

Ashwagandha can also lift your spirits and give you more energy. This plant has active ingredients that can help the body's cells produce energy, therefore enhancing vitality and endurance. Higher energy levels can lead to more satisfying and improved sexual experiences.

The increase in libido caused by ashwagandha has been well researched. According to scientific research, taking Ashwagandha regularly might improve both men's and women's desire for sex. Additionally, by enhancing erections and boosting blood flow to the penis, this herb can help men's erectile function.

The potential of ashwagandha to support healthy hormonal balance may be a crucial element in enhancing sexual performance. The hormone testosterone, which is crucial for both men's and women's desire and sexual health, may be balanced with the aid of this plant. An improved sexual response and more desire may result from a hormonal balance that is ideal.

Ashwagandha is offered in a variety of dosages, including extracts, powders, and capsules. To identify the right dosage and route of ingestion most appropriate for your needs, it is crucial to speak with a health practitioner.

Always get the advice of a medical expert before beginning the use of ashwagandha or any other supplement, particularly if you are on medication or have a history of medical issues. For the best outcomes, a health expert can offer individualized advice on the efficacy and safe usage of this plant.

Yohimbe

An herbaceous plant called yohimbe produces a chemical substance called yohimbine in its bark that is known to have stimulating effects on sexual function. This herb has long been used as a natural aphrodisiac and treatment for increased sexual potency.

Yohimbe bark contains yohimbine, a vasodilator that can widen blood vessels and increase blood flow to the genitalia. Good erection function and heightened sexual sensitivity depend on adequate blood flow. As a result, Yohimbe bark consumption can enhance sexual pleasure and erection function.

Yohimbine, which is present in yohimbe bark, might have negative side effects; thus, it's crucial to utilize it with caution. The most frequent adverse reactions are elevated blood pressure, jitters, anxiety, and sleep difficulties. Yohimbe bark use at high or extended dosages has also been linked to gastrointestinal and cardiac issues.

Prior to using Yohimbe bark or any other product containing Yohimbine, it is imperative to speak with a medical practitioner. People with heart issues, hypertension, sleep disturbances, or other pre-existing medical illnesses should pay particular attention to this. To reduce the risk of side effects, a health expert can evaluate your particular condition, offer tailored information, and propose the right dose.

Yohimbe bark may interfere with various drugs, particularly those used for the treatment of high blood pressure, depression, and cardiac conditions. Before using any product containing Yohimbe bark, it is crucial to let your doctor know about all of your prescription drugs, dietary supplements, and pre-existing medical issues.

Epimedium

The Chinese herb Epimedium, often called Horny Goat Grass, has been used for generations as a natural aphrodisiac. Icariin, a substance found in this plant, has been demonstrated to have positive effects on sexual health.

The capacity of icariin to encourage enhanced blood flow in the vaginal region is one of its key characteristics. To get and keep an erection, enough blood flow is essential. Horny goat grass can assist in boosting blood flow to the erectile tissues, which will enhance men's erectile function. This result can be related to icariin's capacity to inhibit PDE5, an enzyme that lowers blood flow to the vaginal region. Icariin improves vasodilation and boosts blood flow to the corpora cavernosa of the penis by decreasing the activity of this enzyme.

Additionally, horny goat grass can boost the body's synthesis of nitric oxide. A substance called nitric oxide works as a vasodilator to relax muscles and increase blood flow. Nitric oxide production must be enough to encourage blood vessel dilatation and improve blood flow to the vaginal region, which improves erectile function and sexual sensitivity.

Horny goat herb may have positive effects on the neurological system in addition to having an immediate impact on sexual function. The general health and equilibrium of the body may be enhanced by this plant's potential neuroprotective and anti-inflammatory qualities. An uninflamed body and a healthy neural system might encourage improved sexual responsiveness and general wellbeing.

It is crucial to remember that every person may respond differently to the horny goat herb. While some individuals may see positive impacts on their sexual health, others might not experience any appreciable improvement. Before using Horny Goat Grass or any other product to enhance sexual health, it is always advised to speak with a doctor or other healthcare provider. In order to prevent adverse interactions or side effects, this is particularly crucial for those who use drugs or who have pre-existing medical issues.

Even though these herbs are thought to be natural and safe, it is always advised to get the advice of a doctor or herbalist before using them, especially if you are on medication or have a history of medical issues. A health expert will be able to evaluate your particular circumstances and provide you with tailored instructions based on your requirements.

Due to individual differences, each person may react differently to herbal supplements. There can be unfavorable interactions with other drugs or medical conditions, and what works for one person might not work for another. Furthermore, consuming too much of these herbs may have undesirable side effects.

You may obtain a customized treatment plan by consulting with a professional, which will take into consideration your unique requirements and health situation. They may also notify you of any possible contraindications, the proper dose, and any potential adverse effects.

Never undervalue the significance of maintaining responsible, intentional sexual health. Despite the potential advantages these herbs may have, using them safely and effectively requires following medical professionals' recommendations.

Keep in mind that your health is valuable and requires the highest level of care. Before beginning any new therapy or dietary supplement to enhance sexual health, always get the opinion of a trained health expert.

Triya Nanavati

BONUS 3

TYPES OF HERBS TO BE AVOIDED

Several precautions may be taken to prevent herb poisoning, and practically all of them entail utilizing common sense alone. Next, familiarize yourself with plants and their negative effects. If you're planning to go wild, especially, pick up a decent herbal almanac or field guide to the native herbs in your area. By avoiding using a medicine you're unfamiliar with, you can all but assure your own health.

dietary supplements you shouldn't take These items appear like they ought to be harmless. You do use herbs every time you cook, after all. However, some of them might not be free, especially if you take certain medications or have specific medical problems. Before using any supplements, consult your doctor.

Even this well-known vitamin is frequently used to treat anxiety, insomnia, and melancholy. However, it can lead to major health issues like dry mouth, headaches, nausea, and dizziness. Additionally, it could make you susceptible to sunburn. It can also cause problems if you use certain medications, including contraceptive pills, antidepressants, and even cardiac medications. And other chemotherapy treatments might not be as successful.

Safety of supplements These goods seem to be secure. You do use herbs every time you cook, after all. However, some of them might not be free, especially if you take certain medications or have specific medical problems. Before using any supplements, consult your doctor.

John's wort This typical supplement is frequently used for issues with anxiety, insomnia, and depression. However, it may result in negative side effects such as dry mouth, nausea, dizziness, and migraines. Additionally, it can increase your risk of becoming sunburned. Additionally, using some medications, such as birth control pills, antidepressants, and even heart medications, might cause problems. And certain chemotherapy treatments might not work as well.

Kava

This is intended to aid in treating insomnia and anxiety. However, it could harm the liver, like hepatitis. Therefore, if you have kidney or liver issues, you shouldn't take it. If you consume alcohol or use other sedative medications, kava can be deadly as well.

Ginkgo

Many people use this chance to try to sharpen their memory. Numerous people assert that, among other health issues, ginkgo biloba also helps with breathing, brain function, and altitude sickness. However, it could thin your blood and result in bleeding. If you use blood thinners, you should avoid them at all costs.

Arnica Many individuals think that applying this herb's oil to their bodies tends to reduce the discomfort of swelling, pain, and bruises. Others are consuming the supplement in an effort to treat constipation. However, taking the herb might raise blood pressure, quicken the heartbeat, and tighten the chest. It may potentially harm the kidneys, cause a coma, or even cause death.

Goldenseal

This Native American remedy, which has a lengthy history, is used to treat constipation, colds, conjunctivitis, and even cancer. However, the golden seal can alter your heart's rhythm, impact blood clotting, and drop your blood pressure. If you have issues with blood clotting or take blood pressure medications, you should first see your doctor.

Ephedra

This herb, also known as Ma Huang, has been used for thousands of years to treat coughs, nausea, and cold symptoms in China and India. Most recently, it has been employed to assist people in strengthening themselves and losing weight. Nevertheless, research indicates that it may raise the risk of heart issues and strokes, as well as heart rate and blood pressure. Doctors also give warnings about potentially fatal interactions with numerous cardiovascular drugs. Although ephedra has been outlawed as a dietary supplement by the FDA, it is still permitted in some herbal teas.

Ginseng

Some individuals take this in the hopes that it may delay aging. Others use it to treat diabetes, boost immunity, or enhance their sexual performance. However, it may result in a reduction in blood sugar, which may be problematic for those who have diabetes. If you use blood thinners, you should avoid taking them as well.

Black Cohosh

Hot flashes and night sweats are common menopausal symptoms that are treated with this supplement. Women are also attempting to help with PMS. However, anyone with liver issues should avoid it since there is a potential that it might result in inflammation or failure. As more is learned about how they can be affected, those with breast cancer should also be avoided.

Licorice Root

Many people may use it to treat sore throats, bronchitis, stomach ulcers, coughs, and asthma. However, if you have heart trouble, you should first speak with your doctor, as it may raise your blood pressure and affect your heart's rhythm. People with renal conditions may have problems with excessive quantities as well.

Feverfew

The main purpose of this medication is to attempt to avoid migraines. Some people also use it for allergies and rheumatoid arthritis. However, feverfew may interfere with blood coagulation, making it problematic for those who have heart or blood conditions.

Herbs Pregnant Women Should Avoid

Some herbs should not be consumed by expectant mothers. You should exercise special caution while dealing with herbs if you are pregnant, trying to get pregnant, or breastfeeding. Many might result in a miscarriage if consumed. Make sure they are safe before ingesting any herbs by themselves or even just touching them with your bare hands. If in doubt, see your doctor first.

The following are only a handful of the many herbs that could be harmful to expectant mothers.

- Angelica can cause contractions;
- Basil can cause menstruation;

- Black cohosh: can cause pregnancy;
- Catnip: uterine stimulant; may cause contractions;
- Feverfew: can cause menstruation; also affects birth defects;
- Goldenseal: can cause miscarriage;
- Mistletoe: can cause miscarriage;
- Mugwort: will promote menstruation; can also cause miscarriage.
- Call the vet right away if you think your pet may have consumed a hazardous plant.

Plants that could be dangerous for dogs and cats.

Use your magic herbs to stuff poppies, outfit candles, or use them in pouches, but never consume them orally unless you are certain it is okay to do so. Finally, keep in mind that many plants are identified by folk names. When conducting your research and analysis, be sure to review the plants using their scientific names and classifications. Doing so will help ensure that what you are actually looking at and what you think you are looking at are the same thing. herb.

When consumed in excess, buckeye can cause muscular tremors and epilepsy in both dogs and cats. It can also cause vomiting and diarrhea.

Chamomile may make dogs and cats throw up and have diarrhea. Foxglove: In cats and dogs, it can cause arrhythmias, an abnormally rapid heart rate, and even death.

Holly berries can make dogs and cats vomit, slobber, and shake their heads.

Jimson weed can cause dilated pupils, nervousness, light sensitivity, and anxiety in bigger animals like horses and cattle, in addition to cats and dogs.

Mistletoe berries can make dogs and cats drool, feel queasy, have diarrhea, and have stomach aches. Death can result from consuming too much.

Although the dried leaves of the pennyroyal plant are often benign, ingesting the essential oil can cause liver failure. Female animals have also demonstrated miscarriage.

For both cats and dogs, tobacco use can result in mild to severe vomiting, an elevated or atypical heart rate and breathing, overstimulation, paralysis, or even death.

BONUS 4

HERBS FOR FACIAL CARE

Natural Facial Care with Basil Ocimum basilicum, a mild astringent found in basil, is an excellent skin toner and moisturizer. Their anti-inflammatory and anti-bacterial properties help with a number of skin issues, including wrinkles. Basil's high antioxidant content, which prevents free radicals from damaging skin cells, accounts for its long history of usage as an anti-aging remedy.

Toner, mature skin, acne, and oily skin are all benefits.

Burdock

Burdock, Arctium lappa, has been used for many years to treat many kinds of chronic skin issues because it is rich in fatty acids that encourage blood flow, enhance blood supply, and eliminate pollutants. The root is a superb herb for acne and a natural acne treatment due to its anti-inflammatory and antibacterial qualities. Good for: acne; skin irritation

Calendula Natural

The calming, anti-inflammatory, and healing properties of calendula officinalis assist in lessening skin irritation and swelling in those with sensitive and eczema-prone skin. It nourishes and softens the skin while being effective in the treatment of rashes, irritated skin, eczema, acne, and sunburn.

Good for: Irritated Skin; Astringent/Toner

Chamomile Natural

With its emollient, therapeutic, tonic, antioxidant, and anti-inflammatory characteristics, chamomile, Matricaria recutita, has a calming and soothing impact on injured skin. It contains blueene, which reduces puffiness and clears dirt from pores. The tension headache, pressure, and chest tightness brought on by congestion may also be relieved with the help of chamomile when used as face steam.

Great for dry hair, irritated skin, congestion, and chamomile astringent or toner.

Chickweed Natural

Chickweed, Stellaria press, offers relief from chronic itching brought on by eczema, psoriasis, and other rashes and is useful in the treatment of inflammatory skin diseases. Chickweed salve hydrates skin that is dry or damaged. Excellent for itchy hair and irritated skin.

Dandelion Natural Skin Care Acne Dandelion

The root of Taraxacum officinale aids in the body's elimination of excessive hair bacteria. The root, which is a high source of vitamins A, B, C, and D as well as trace minerals, encourages clean skin and is excellent for treating skin conditions like acne. For the treatment of eczema and other skin problems, it is administered topically. It's ideal for: dandelions Irritated Hair: Acne

Elder Flowers

The first plant cultivated by humans was Sambucus nigra. They are somewhat astringent and aid in soothing dry, aging skin. The fading of freckles, age spots, and other facial imperfections has been achieved with elderflower tea. For thousands of years, elder blossoms have been used to cure skin irritation. beneficial for older skin, acne,

Clean Herbal Facial Scrub

Herbal, Natural Scrub Approximately once or twice per week, it can enhance drainage and help remove dead skin cells. The herbal scrub's exfoliating effect makes the skin on the face feel smooth and beautiful. If you have sensitive skin, exercise particular care. Overly rigorous scrubbing may leave ugly spots, which will eventually disappear. If you have sensitive skin, exercise particular care.

Ingredients: oat flour, 1 cup (choose one or use a combination). 1/3 cup dry powdered herbs 1 tablespoon of bittersweet sugar Directions Use a pristine coffee grinder to grind herbs.

Oat flour, spices, and sugar are combined in a very clean container or basin. For two or three months, the scrub can be stored in a container with a tight seal in a cool, dry environment. Put a tiny amount of the scrub in the palm of your hand. To produce a paste, add just enough water. While avoiding your eyes, evenly spread the paste mixture across your face. Make gentle circular motions on your skin. Okay, give it a good rinse.

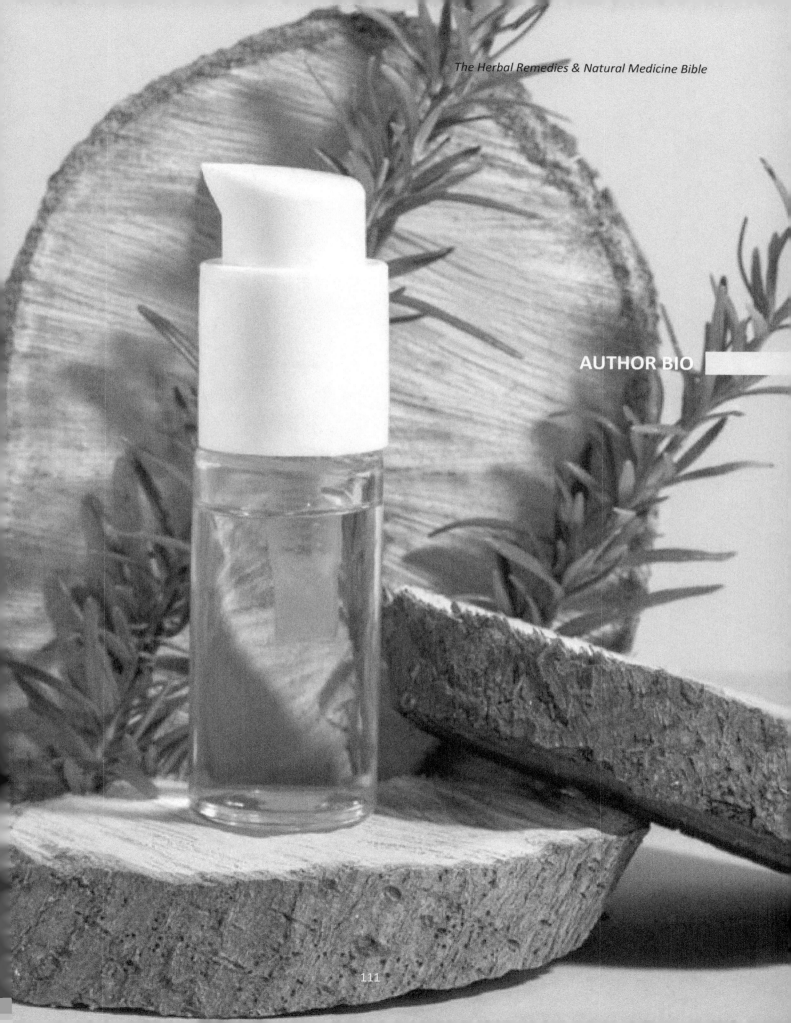

AUTHOR BIO

Triya Nanavati

Triya Nanavati

Triya Nanavati is a renowned expert in the field of herbal remedies and natural medicine, with a deep passion for holistic healing. With extensive knowledge and years of experience, she has become a trusted authority in the industry. Triya's expertise lies in exploring the healing properties of plants and natural ingredients, as well as their traditional uses in different cultures around the world.

Triya's journey into herbal remedies began with a personal health challenge that led her to seek alternative and natural solutions. She delved into ancient texts, researched traditional healing practices, and studied to expand her understanding of the subject.

She advocates for a holistic approach that considers the physical, emotional, and spiritual aspects of health. She also emphasizes the importance of lifestyle choices, nutrition, and mindfulness practices to support overall well-being.

Made in the USA
Monee, IL
18 November 2023

45935770R00066